Harmony of Healing: Exploring the World of Alternative & Holistic Medicine

Welcome to the world of alternative and holistic medicine, where healing is viewed as a harmonious integration of mind, body, and spirit. In "Harmony of Healing: Exploring the World of Alternative & Holistic Medicine," we embark on a journey to discover the diverse and ancient practices that have been empowering individuals to achieve optimal well-being for centuries.

In our modern world, the demand for alternative and holistic approaches to health and wellness is steadily growing. People are seeking comprehensive and natural solutions that complement traditional medical treatments and focus on the root causes of health issues rather than merely treating symptoms. This book is a comprehensive guide that delves into the various disciplines of alternative and holistic medicine, shedding light on their principles, benefits, and applications.

We will explore the practices of naturopathy, where nature's healing power is harnessed to restore balance and vitality within the body. Acupuncture, an ancient Chinese therapy, will be unveiled, revealing its efficacy in promoting energy flow and relieving pain. Chiropractic, a holistic approach to spinal health, will be explored as we understand its role in aligning the body's musculoskeletal structure for overall wellness.

Delving into diet therapy, we will understand how the food we consume can be harnessed as medicine to prevent and treat various ailments. Holistic medicine, a philosophy that embraces the interconnectedness of mind, body, and spirit, will be uncovered, offering a comprehensive approach to health that considers all aspects of an individual's well-being.

We will journey into the realm of hypnotherapy, where the power of the mind is harnessed to transform behaviors and beliefs. Mind-body medicine, also known as psychoneuroimmunology, will be explored as we delve into the fascinating connection between mental and physical health. Lastly, we will unveil osteopathy, a gentle and hands-on approach to healing that focuses on the body's natural ability to self-regulate and heal.

Throughout this book, we will emphasize the importance of embracing a holistic perspective on health, recognizing that true well-being extends beyond physical health to encompass mental, emotional, and spiritual aspects. By exploring these various disciplines, we aim to empower readers with the knowledge and understanding to make informed decisions about their health, embracing a harmony of healing that is grounded in natural, time-tested wisdom.

Join us on this enlightening journey as we unravel the rich tapestry of alternative and holistic medicine, where ancient traditions and modern science converge to foster a balanced and harmonious approach to health and wellness. Let us embark together on a path towards empowerment and self-discovery, as we unlock the boundless potential of a life lived in harmony with the principles of alternative and holistic medicine.

I. Introduction

- The rise of Alternative & Holistic Medicine

II. Naturopathy

- Principles and philosophy of naturopathic medicine
- Treatment modalities: herbal medicine, homeopathy, hydrotherapy, etc.
- The role of nutrition and lifestyle in naturopathy

III. Acupuncture

- History and principles of acupuncture
- Meridians and energy flow in Traditional Chinese Medicine
- Acupuncture techniques and practices
- Efficacy of acupuncture in treating various conditions

IV. Chiropractic

- Understanding the concept of spinal alignment and nervous system
- Techniques and adjustments in chiropractic care
- Conditions treated by chiropractors
- Integrating chiropractic with other holistic approaches

V. Diet Therapy

- Role of diet in promoting health and preventing diseases
- The impact of different food groups on the body
- Specific diets for various health conditions
- Incorporating nutrition into holistic treatment plans

VI. Holistic Medicine

- Holistic approach to healthcare and wellness
- Integrating mind, body, and spirit in treatment
- The role of complementary therapies in holistic medicine
- Holistic healing techniques and practices

VII. Hypnotherapy

- Understanding the power of the subconscious mind
- Inducing hypnosis and guiding clients through therapy
- Applications of hypnotherapy in stress reduction, pain management, etc.
- Ethical considerations in hypnotherapy practice

VIII. Mind-Body Medicine (Psychoneuroimmunology)

- The mind-body connection in health and disease
- Techniques for managing stress and improving mental health
- Psychoneuroimmunology and its impact on the immune system
- Mindfulness and meditation practices

IX. Osteopathy

- Principles and philosophy of osteopathic medicine
- Osteopathic manipulative techniques and bodywork

- Conditions treated by osteopaths
- Integrating osteopathy with other alternative therapies

X. Integrative Medicine

- The importance of collaboration between conventional and alternative medicine
- The rise of integrative medical centers and clinics
- Case studies showcasing successful integration of modalities
- Future trends in alternative and holistic medicine

XI. Conclusion

- Recap of key insights and learnings
- Emphasizing the value of Alternative & Holistic Medicine in modern healthcare
- Encouragement to explore and embrace alternative approaches to health and healing

The rise of Alternative & Holistic Medicine

The rise of alternative and holistic medicine is a notable trend in the field of healthcare. Traditional medicine, often referred to as conventional or allopathic medicine, has long been the dominant approach to healthcare in many parts of the world. However, in recent years, there has been a growing interest and acceptance of alternative and holistic practices as complementary or alternative options to conventional medicine.

Alternative medicine encompasses a wide range of therapies and practices that are not part of mainstream medical care. Some of the most popular forms of alternative medicine include herbal medicine, acupuncture, chiropractic care, homeopathy, naturopathy, and traditional Chinese medicine, among others. These practices often focus on treating the whole person, including their physical, emotional, and spiritual well-being, and may use natural remedies or non-invasive methods.

Holistic medicine, on the other hand, is an approach that considers the whole person in the context of their environment and seeks to address the root causes of health issues, rather than just treating the symptoms. Holistic practitioners may incorporate a combination of conventional and alternative therapies to provide comprehensive care for their patients.

Several factors have contributed to the rise of alternative and holistic medicine:

    1. Patient Demand: Many people are seeking more

personalized and natural approaches to healthcare. They may be dissatisfied with the side effects or limitations of conventional treatments or may be looking for ways to improve their overall well-being beyond just addressing specific symptoms.

2. Increasing Research and Evidence: As interest in alternative and holistic therapies grows, there is a greater focus on scientific research to validate their effectiveness. Some alternative practices have shown promising results in clinical studies, leading to increased acceptance among healthcare professionals and the public.

3. Integrative Medicine: Some healthcare institutions and clinics are adopting an integrative medicine approach, which combines both conventional and alternative therapies to provide a more comprehensive and patient-centered approach to care.

4. Global Influence: Traditional healing practices from different cultures have gained recognition and acceptance in various parts of the world, leading to a more diverse and inclusive approach to healthcare.

5. Wellness and Prevention: Many alternative and holistic practices emphasize preventive care and wellness promotion, aligning with the increasing focus on maintaining good health and preventing chronic diseases.

6. Internet and Information Access: The internet has provided a platform for individuals to access information about alternative and holistic medicine, empowering them to make informed choices about their healthcare.

It's essential to note that while some alternative and holistic practices have gained popularity, not all of them have been scientifically validated, and some may lack sufficient evidence of efficacy. As with any form of healthcare, it is crucial for individuals to consult qualified healthcare professionals and make informed decisions about their treatment options.

The rise of alternative and holistic medicine reflects a broader shift towards more patient-centered and comprehensive approaches to health and wellness. As the field continues to evolve, there is ongoing dialogue and research to explore how these practices can best be integrated into mainstream healthcare to benefit patients and promote overall well-being.

Naturopathy

Naturopathy is a form of alternative medicine that emphasizes the body's natural ability to heal itself and focuses on promoting overall health and well-being. Naturopathic medicine practitioners use a combination of traditional healing methods, natural therapies, and evidence-based medicine to treat and prevent illness. The practice is based on the principles of holistic health, individualized treatment, and the belief that the body has an innate ability to heal when provided with the right conditions.

Key principles of naturopathy include:

1. The Healing Power of Nature: Naturopaths believe that the body has an inherent ability to heal itself when given the right support. They focus on enhancing the body's natural healing processes rather than merely suppressing symptoms.
2. Identify and Treat the Root Cause: Naturopaths aim to identify and address the underlying causes of illness rather than just treating the symptoms. This approach is designed to promote long-term health and prevent the recurrence of health issues.
3. First, Do No Harm: Naturopaths prioritize using non-invasive and low-risk treatments to minimize the potential for harmful side effects.
4. Treat the Whole Person: Naturopaths consider all aspects of a person's health, including physical, mental, emotional, and spiritual well-being. They take into account the individual's lifestyle, genetics, and environmental factors when creating a treatment plan.
5. Education and Prevention: Naturopaths emphasize

patient education and work to empower individuals to take an active role in their health. They also focus on preventive measures to promote overall wellness and reduce the risk of future health problems.

Naturopathic treatments may include:

- Herbal medicine: The use of plants and plant extracts to support healing and treat various health conditions.
- Nutrition and dietary counseling: Customized dietary plans to address specific health concerns and promote optimal nutrition.
- Lifestyle modifications: Guidance on adopting healthy lifestyle habits such as exercise, stress management, and sleep hygiene.
- Homeopathy: The use of highly diluted substances to stimulate the body's healing responses.
- Hydrotherapy: The therapeutic use of water in various forms, such as hot and cold compresses or baths.
- Physical manipulation: Techniques like massage, chiropractic adjustments, and bodywork to promote musculoskeletal health.
- Counseling and mind-body approaches: Techniques to address emotional and mental health issues that may impact physical well-being.

It's essential to note that naturopathy is a complementary approach to healthcare and is not intended to replace conventional medical treatments for serious medical conditions. Naturopaths work alongside other healthcare professionals and may collaborate with medical doctors to provide integrative care.

As with any form of healthcare, individuals considering naturopathy should seek guidance from qualified and licensed naturopathic practitioners. Naturopaths in many countries undergo extensive training and are regulated by professional organizations to ensure ethical practice and patient safety.

Principles and philosophy of naturopathic medicine

The principles and philosophy of naturopathic medicine are rooted in the belief that the body has an inherent ability to heal itself and that the role of a healthcare provider is to support and facilitate the body's natural healing processes. Naturopathic medicine is based on a holistic approach to health, recognizing that physical, mental, emotional, and spiritual aspects are interconnected and play a vital role in overall well-being.

The principles of naturopathic medicine include:

1. Vis Medicatrix Naturae - The Healing Power of Nature: Naturopathic medicine acknowledges the body's innate ability to heal and restore balance when given the right conditions. The focus is on supporting and strengthening the body's healing processes rather than suppressing symptoms.

2. Tolle Causam - Identify and Treat the Root Cause: Naturopathic practitioners seek to identify and address the underlying causes of illness rather than solely treating the symptoms. By addressing the root cause, the goal is to promote long-term health and prevent the recurrence of health issues.

3. Primum Non Nocere - First, Do No Harm: Naturopathic treatments aim to use the least invasive and least harmful therapies to avoid causing further harm to the patient. The emphasis is on safe and effective treatments with minimal side effects.

4. Docere - Doctor as Teacher: Naturopathic physicians act as educators, empowering patients to take an active role in their health. They provide information and guidance to help patients understand their health conditions and make informed decisions about their care.

5. Treat the Whole Person - Tolle Totum: Naturopathic medicine considers the whole person, taking into account physical, mental, emotional, and spiritual aspects of health. The focus is on addressing the individual's unique health needs and circumstances.

6. Prevention - Praevenire: Naturopathic medicine emphasizes preventive measures to promote overall health and well-being. Through education and lifestyle modifications, naturopathic practitioners aim to prevent the onset of illness and disease.

7. Establish Health and Wellness - Salutogenesis: Naturopathic medicine strives not only to treat illness but also to optimize health and wellness. The goal is to help individuals achieve their highest potential for well-being.

Naturopathic physicians use a wide range of therapies and treatments, including herbal medicine, nutrition and dietary counseling, homeopathy, hydrotherapy, physical manipulation, mind-body techniques, and lifestyle counseling. They may also integrate conventional medical treatments when necessary, working collaboratively with other healthcare providers to provide comprehensive care.

Naturopathic medicine places a strong emphasis on the individualized approach to patient care, recognizing that each person's health needs are unique. Naturopaths take the time to listen to their patients, understand their health history, and tailor treatment plans accordingly. They also focus on patient education, empowering individuals to make informed decisions about their health and lifestyle choices.

It's important to note that naturopathic medicine is regulated differently in various countries, and the scope of practice may vary. When seeking naturopathic care, it's essential to ensure that the practitioner is licensed and trained according to the regulations of the relevant governing body in the respective country.

Treatment modalities: herbal medicine, homeopathy, hydrotherapy, etc.

Treatment modalities in naturopathic medicine encompass a wide range of natural therapies and approaches that aim to support the body's innate healing abilities and promote overall well-being. These modalities are used in conjunction with individualized treatment plans to address the root cause of health issues and restore balance in the body. Some of the key treatment modalities in naturopathic medicine include:

1. Herbal Medicine: Herbal medicine involves the use of plant-based remedies, such as tinctures, teas, extracts, and powders, to support the body's healing processes. Different herbs are chosen based on their specific medicinal properties and their ability to address the individual's health needs.

2. Homeopathy: Homeopathy is a system of medicine based on the principle of "like cures like," where a substance that produces symptoms in a healthy person is used to treat similar symptoms in a sick person. Homeopathic remedies are highly diluted and work on an energetic level to stimulate the body's self-healing mechanisms.

3. Hydrotherapy: Hydrotherapy uses water in various forms, such as baths, compresses, and steam, to promote healing and improve circulation. Hydrotherapy can help with pain relief, relaxation, and detoxification.

4. Nutrition and Dietary Counseling: Naturopathic

practitioners provide personalized dietary recommendations to address specific health concerns and optimize nutrition. Nutritional counseling may include guidance on specific foods, dietary supplements, and lifestyle modifications.

5. Lifestyle Counseling: Lifestyle counseling involves working with patients to identify and modify lifestyle factors that may be contributing to health issues. This may include stress management, sleep hygiene, exercise, and other lifestyle adjustments.

6. Physical Manipulation: Physical manipulation techniques, such as massage, chiropractic adjustments, and bodywork, are used to address musculoskeletal imbalances and promote physical well-being.

7. Mind-Body Techniques: Mind-body approaches, including meditation, relaxation techniques, and counseling, are utilized to support emotional and mental health and their impact on physical well-being.

8. Acupuncture: Acupuncture is an ancient Chinese therapy that involves inserting thin needles into specific points on the body to stimulate energy flow and promote balance.

9. Counseling and Stress Management: Counseling may involve talk therapy and cognitive-behavioral techniques to address emotional and psychological factors that may be influencing health.

10. Physical Therapies: Some naturopathic practitioners may use physical therapies such as heat therapy, cold therapy, and therapeutic exercises to support healing and recovery.

11. Energy Therapies: Energy-based therapies, such as Reiki and therapeutic touch, are used to balance the body's energy fields and promote healing.

It's important to note that the use of these treatment modalities varies among naturopathic practitioners and is tailored to the individual needs and preferences of each patient. Naturopathic treatments are typically selected based on the patient's health history, current health status, and specific health goals.

If considering naturopathic treatments, it is advisable to consult with a qualified and licensed naturopathic physician who can provide personalized care and ensure safe and effective use of these therapies. Naturopathic medicine is complementary to conventional medical care and can work alongside other healthcare approaches when needed.

The role of nutrition and lifestyle in naturopathy

Nutrition and lifestyle play a fundamental role in naturopathic medicine. Naturopathic practitioners recognize that what we eat, how we live, and the environment we are exposed to have a profound impact on our overall health and well-being. The integration of nutrition and lifestyle interventions is central to the naturopathic approach, as these factors are essential in supporting the body's natural healing processes and preventing illness.

1. Individualized Nutrition: Naturopathic physicians take a personalized approach to nutrition, considering each individual's unique dietary needs, health conditions, and goals. They may recommend specific foods, dietary patterns, and supplements to address deficiencies, support organ function, and promote optimal health.

2. Nutritional Counseling: Naturopathic practitioners provide guidance and education on healthy eating habits and lifestyle choices. They empower patients to make informed decisions about their diet and encourage the adoption of sustainable dietary practices.

3. Prevention and Wellness: Naturopathic medicine places a strong emphasis on preventive care. Nutrition and lifestyle interventions are used proactively to prevent the development of chronic diseases and promote overall wellness.

4. Addressing Nutritional Deficiencies: Naturopathic physicians assess for nutritional deficiencies that may

contribute to health issues. They may use laboratory tests and dietary analysis to identify specific nutrient imbalances and provide targeted interventions.

5. Weight Management: Naturopathic medicine recognizes the importance of maintaining a healthy weight for overall health. Practitioners may provide personalized weight management plans that include dietary modifications, exercise recommendations, and lifestyle changes.

6. Gut Health: Naturopaths focus on the health of the gastrointestinal system, as it plays a crucial role in nutrient absorption, immune function, and overall well-being. They may use dietary interventions and probiotics to support gut health.

7. Lifestyle Modifications: Naturopathic medicine recognizes the impact of lifestyle choices on health outcomes. Naturopathic practitioners may provide guidance on stress management, sleep hygiene, exercise, and other lifestyle modifications to enhance overall health.

8. Integrative Approach: Naturopathic physicians work collaboratively with other healthcare providers, including conventional medical professionals, to integrate nutrition and lifestyle interventions into comprehensive treatment plans.

9. Disease Management: In addition to preventive care, nutrition and lifestyle interventions are utilized to manage chronic conditions and support individuals with chronic illnesses.

10. Detoxification: Naturopathic medicine may incorporate detoxification protocols to support the body's natural detoxification pathways and eliminate toxins that may negatively impact health.

By emphasizing the importance of nutrition and lifestyle, naturopathic medicine seeks to empower individuals to take an active role in their health and make positive changes that contribute to their overall well-being. These holistic approaches are designed to complement conventional medical care and provide a comprehensive and individualized approach to health and healing. It's essential to consult with a qualified naturopathic physician to receive personalized guidance and recommendations based on individual health needs and goals.

Acupuncture

Acupuncture is a key component of traditional Chinese medicine (TCM) and is a therapeutic technique that involves the insertion of thin, sterile needles into specific points on the body. The goal of acupuncture is to restore the flow of energy (referred to as "Qi" or "Chi") along meridians or pathways in the body. By doing so, acupuncture aims to balance the body's energy, promote healing, and improve overall health and well-being.

Principles of Acupuncture:

1. Qi and Meridians: According to TCM principles, Qi is the vital life force that flows through meridians, which are pathways in the body. When the flow of Qi is disrupted or blocked, it can lead to imbalances and health issues.
2. Yin and Yang: TCM emphasizes the balance between opposing forces known as Yin and Yang. Health is believed to be achieved when there is harmony and balance between these forces.
3. Acupuncture Points: Acupuncture points are specific locations on the body where needles are inserted to access and influence the flow of Qi along the meridians.

How Acupuncture Works:

Acupuncture is thought to stimulate the body's natural healing mechanisms by promoting the release of neurotransmitters, endorphins, and other biochemical substances. These substances help reduce pain, inflammation, and stress while enhancing overall well-being.

The Acupuncture Procedure:

During an acupuncture session, a licensed acupuncturist inserts thin, sterile needles into specific acupuncture points on the body. The needles are left in place for a certain period, typically 15-30 minutes, during which the individual may experience sensations like warmth, tingling, or a dull ache. The treatment is generally well-tolerated and is known to be relatively painless.

Conditions Treated with Acupuncture:

Acupuncture has been used to address a wide range of health conditions, including:

1. Pain Management: Acupuncture is often sought for the relief of chronic pain conditions, such as back pain, migraines, arthritis, and musculoskeletal injuries.
2. Stress and Anxiety: Many individuals use acupuncture as a complementary approach to reduce stress, anxiety, and promote relaxation.
3. Digestive Disorders: Acupuncture can be beneficial in managing conditions like irritable bowel syndrome (IBS), acid reflux, and nausea.
4. Women's Health: Acupuncture is sometimes used to address menstrual irregularities, fertility issues, and menopausal symptoms.
5. Respiratory Conditions: Some people turn to acupuncture for support in managing asthma, allergies, and sinusitis.
6. Mental Health: Acupuncture may be utilized to complement conventional therapies for conditions such as depression and post-traumatic stress disorder (PTSD).

Acupuncture Safety:

When performed by a trained and licensed practitioner, acupuncture is considered a safe and low-risk treatment. The use of sterile needles and adherence to safety guidelines help minimize the risk of adverse effects.

It's essential to consult with a qualified acupuncturist to discuss your specific health concerns and to determine if acupuncture is a suitable treatment option for you. Acupuncture should not be used as a replacement for conventional medical care, especially in serious or life-threatening conditions, but rather as a complementary therapy to enhance overall health and well-being.

History and principles of acupuncture

History of Acupuncture:

Acupuncture has a long and rich history that dates back over 2,000 years. It originated in ancient China and is one of the key components of traditional Chinese medicine (TCM). The practice of acupuncture was first documented in the classic Chinese medical text "Huangdi Neijing" or "The Yellow Emperor's Classic of Internal Medicine," which is believed to have been compiled around the 2nd century BCE.

Over the centuries, acupuncture techniques and theories evolved and were refined. Acupuncture spread to neighboring countries and regions, including Japan, Korea, and other parts of East Asia, where it integrated with local healing traditions.

Principles of Acupuncture:

Acupuncture is based on several fundamental principles that are core to traditional Chinese medicine:

1. Qi (Chi) and Meridians: Central to acupuncture is the concept of Qi, the vital life force that flows through the body's meridians or energy pathways. The meridians are channels that connect the body's organs and tissues, and the free flow of Qi along these meridians is essential for maintaining health.
2. Yin and Yang: In TCM, health is achieved when there is a balance between the opposing forces of Yin and Yang. Yin represents qualities like darkness, coolness, and rest, while Yang represents qualities like brightness, warmth, and activity. Imbalances between Yin and Yang

are thought to contribute to illness and disease.

3. Acupuncture Points: Acupuncture points are specific locations on the body where needles are inserted to access and influence the flow of Qi along the meridians. There are hundreds of acupuncture points throughout the body, each associated with different organs and functions.

4. Blockages and Imbalances: Illness and pain are believed to result from blockages or imbalances in the flow of Qi. Acupuncture aims to restore the proper flow of Qi and balance Yin and Yang to promote healing.

5. Individualized Treatment: Each person is considered unique in TCM, and the diagnosis and treatment are tailored to the individual's specific patterns of imbalance and health concerns.

Acupuncture Techniques:

Acupuncture techniques involve the insertion of thin, sterile needles into acupuncture points on the body. The needles are typically left in place for a short period, during which the patient may experience sensations like warmth, tingling, or a dull ache.

Other techniques used in acupuncture include:

- Moxibustion: The burning of dried mugwort (moxa) near acupuncture points to warm and stimulate them.
- Cupping: The application of glass or plastic cups to the skin to create a vacuum, promoting blood flow and relieving muscle tension.
- Electroacupuncture: A technique where a small electric current is passed through the acupuncture needles to enhance the treatment's effects.

Modern Acupuncture:

In modern times, acupuncture has gained recognition and popularity worldwide. It is often used as a complementary therapy alongside conventional medicine to address various health conditions and promote overall well-being. Acupuncture is now practiced by licensed acupuncturists and practitioners trained in traditional Chinese medicine, as well as by healthcare professionals in other disciplines who have received specialized acupuncture training.

The principles and techniques of acupuncture continue to be studied and researched, and acupuncture is increasingly integrated into mainstream healthcare settings as a safe and effective complementary therapy.

Meridians and energy flow in Traditional Chinese Medicine

In Traditional Chinese Medicine (TCM), meridians and energy flow are central concepts that form the foundation of the diagnostic and treatment principles. According to TCM theory, the body's vital energy, known as "Qi" (pronounced chee), flows through a network of meridians or channels. These meridians are pathways that connect different parts of the body, including organs, tissues, and physiological systems.

Key Elements of Meridians and Energy Flow in TCM:

1. Qi (Chi): Qi is the fundamental life force or vital energy that sustains all living beings. It is believed to flow through the meridians and nourish the body's organs and tissues. The balanced and harmonious flow of Qi is essential for maintaining health and well-being.

2. Yin and Yang: The concept of Yin and Yang is fundamental to TCM and the understanding of energy flow. Yin and Yang are opposing yet complementary forces that exist in all aspects of life. Yin represents qualities like darkness, coolness, and rest, while Yang represents qualities like brightness, warmth, and activity. Health is achieved when there is a balance between Yin and Yang in the body.

3. Meridians: There are twelve main meridians in TCM, each associated with specific organs and their related functions. Six of these meridians are classified as Yin, and the other six as Yang. The meridians are named

after the organs they are associated with, such as the Liver meridian, Heart meridian, Lung meridian, etc.

4. Acupuncture Points: Along the meridians, there are specific points called acupuncture points or acupoints. These points are where the flow of Qi can be accessed and influenced. By inserting thin, sterile needles into these acupoints, an acupuncturist can adjust the flow of Qi and restore balance in the body.

5. Energy Blockages and Imbalances: Health issues are thought to arise when there are blockages or imbalances in the flow of Qi through the meridians. Blockages can lead to symptoms and discomfort, while imbalances can manifest as excess or deficiency of Qi in certain areas.

6. Energy Circulation: In TCM, the flow of Qi is not static but dynamic, constantly circulating throughout the meridians. The circulation of Qi helps to maintain the body's functions and adapt to changes in the internal and external environment.

Treatment with Acupuncture:

In acupuncture, the insertion of needles at specific acupoints is aimed at restoring the balanced flow of Qi through the meridians. By addressing the underlying imbalances or blockages, the body's natural healing mechanisms are activated, promoting relief from symptoms and supporting overall health.

While the concept of meridians and energy flow is central to TCM, it differs from the perspective of Western medicine. Scientific research into the existence and mechanisms of Qi and meridians is ongoing, and acupuncture is increasingly studied for its clinical efficacy and mechanisms of action. Nonetheless, acupuncture remains a valued and widely used form of complementary therapy that has been practiced for centuries in the context of TCM principles.

Acupuncture techniques and practices

Acupuncture is a traditional healing technique that involves the insertion of thin, sterile needles into specific points on the body known as acupuncture points or acupoints. These needles are typically left in place for a short duration, and the practice aims to promote the flow of vital energy (Qi) along the body's meridians, restore balance, and alleviate various health conditions. In addition to traditional acupuncture, other acupuncture techniques and related practices have been developed over time. Here are some common acupuncture techniques and practices:

1. Traditional Acupuncture: This is the most common form of acupuncture, where fine needles are inserted into acupoints to stimulate the flow of Qi and restore balance in the body.
2. Electroacupuncture: In this technique, a small electrical current is applied to the acupuncture needles to enhance the effects of the treatment. It is often used for conditions that require stronger stimulation.
3. Moxibustion: Moxibustion involves burning dried mugwort (moxa) near or on the skin at acupoints to warm and stimulate the flow of Qi. Direct moxibustion involves placing a small cone of moxa on an acupoint and lighting it, while indirect moxibustion uses a moxa stick held close to the skin.
4. Cupping: Cupping involves placing glass, bamboo, or plastic cups on the skin and creating a vacuum by suction. This technique promotes blood flow, relieves muscle tension, and is commonly used for pain relief.
5. Acupressure: Acupressure is a non-invasive technique

that involves applying pressure to acupoints with fingers, thumbs, or other devices instead of using needles. It is often used as a self-help technique for pain relief and stress reduction.

6. Scalp Acupuncture: This technique involves inserting very fine needles into specific scalp areas corresponding to the affected body parts or organs. It is commonly used for neurological conditions and motor function disorders.

7. Auricular Acupuncture: Also known as ear acupuncture, this technique involves stimulating specific points on the ear that correspond to different organs and body parts. It is often used for addiction treatment and pain management.

8. Korean Hand Acupuncture: This technique focuses on the acupoints on the hands, which are believed to be microsystems of the whole body. It is used for various health issues and is particularly popular in Korean traditional medicine.

9. Five Element Acupuncture: Based on the principles of the Five Elements theory (Wood, Fire, Earth, Metal, Water), this approach considers an individual's constitutional type and treats imbalances related to the elements.

10. Laser Acupuncture: Instead of using needles, low-level laser beams are applied to acupoints to stimulate the flow of Qi. It is a non-invasive technique often used for those who are needle-phobic or sensitive to needles.

Acupuncture is commonly used to address a wide range of health issues, including pain management, stress reduction, digestive disorders, respiratory conditions, and more. It is important to seek acupuncture services from qualified and licensed practitioners who have received proper training in acupuncture techniques and safety practices.

Efficacy of acupuncture in treating various conditions

Acupuncture has been studied extensively for its efficacy in treating various health conditions, and research has shown promising results for a wide range of ailments. While the effectiveness of acupuncture can vary from individual to individual and may not be a stand-alone solution for all conditions, it is considered safe and often used as a complementary therapy alongside conventional medical treatments. Here are some conditions for which acupuncture has shown potential efficacy:

1. Pain Management: Acupuncture is widely recognized for its effectiveness in relieving pain. It is commonly used to treat chronic pain conditions, such as lower back pain, osteoarthritis, migraines, and headaches.
2. Musculoskeletal Disorders: Acupuncture has been shown to improve mobility and function in individuals with conditions like knee osteoarthritis, neck pain, and fibromyalgia.
3. Nausea and Vomiting: Acupuncture is often used in cancer patients undergoing chemotherapy or postoperative patients to reduce nausea and vomiting.
4. Anxiety and Stress: Acupuncture may help reduce symptoms of anxiety and stress and promote relaxation.
5. Insomnia: Acupuncture may improve sleep quality and help with insomnia.
6. Digestive Disorders: Acupuncture has shown potential

in alleviating symptoms of irritable bowel syndrome (IBS), indigestion, and constipation.

7. Menstrual and Menopausal Symptoms: Acupuncture may help manage symptoms associated with menstrual disorders and menopause, such as menstrual pain, hot flashes, and mood swings.

8. Respiratory Conditions: Acupuncture has been studied for its potential benefits in asthma management and improving symptoms in chronic obstructive pulmonary disease (COPD) patients.

9. Allergies: Some studies suggest that acupuncture may help alleviate allergy symptoms, such as nasal congestion and itching.

10. Fertility and Reproductive Health: Acupuncture may be used in conjunction with assisted reproductive technologies to improve fertility outcomes and support overall reproductive health.

It's important to note that while acupuncture has shown promise in these areas, it is not a replacement for conventional medical treatments. Always consult with a qualified healthcare professional before incorporating acupuncture or any complementary therapy into your treatment plan.

The efficacy of acupuncture can also depend on the individual's response to treatment, the expertise of the acupuncturist, and the frequency and duration of treatment sessions. As with any medical intervention, results may vary, and it's essential to work with a licensed and experienced acupuncturist for the best possible outcomes.

Chiropractic

Chiropractic is a healthcare profession that focuses on diagnosing and treating musculoskeletal and nervous system disorders, particularly those related to the spine. Chiropractors use hands-on spinal manipulation and other manual therapies to restore proper alignment and mobility of the spine, aiming to alleviate pain, improve function, and support the body's natural ability to heal itself.

Principles and Philosophy of Chiropractic:

- The fundamental principle of chiropractic is that the body's structure, particularly the spine, plays a crucial role in overall health. Chiropractors believe that misalignments or subluxations in the spine can interfere with the nervous system's function, leading to various health issues.
- Chiropractic care is based on the concept that the body has an innate ability to heal itself, and by correcting spinal misalignments, the body's natural healing processes can be enhanced.
- Chiropractors emphasize a holistic approach to healthcare, considering the whole person rather than just focusing on specific symptoms or conditions.

Chiropractic Treatment Techniques:

- Spinal Adjustment: This is the primary treatment method used by chiropractors. It involves the application of controlled force to specific joints of the spine or other parts of the body to correct misalignments and restore proper movement.

- Mobilization: This technique involves the manual manipulation of joints to improve range of motion and reduce pain.
- Soft Tissue Techniques: Chiropractors may use massage, stretching, and other manual therapies to address soft tissue injuries and muscle tension.
- Exercise and Rehabilitation: Chiropractors often prescribe exercises and stretches to strengthen muscles, improve flexibility, and support the treatment of musculoskeletal issues.
- Lifestyle Counseling: Chiropractors may provide advice on nutrition, ergonomics, and other lifestyle factors to promote overall well-being.

Conditions Treated by Chiropractors: Chiropractic care is commonly used to treat a variety of conditions, including:

- Back pain and neck pain
- Headaches and migraines
- Joint pain, such as in the shoulders, knees, and hips
- Sciatica
- Whiplash and other injuries from accidents or trauma
- Arthritis and other degenerative joint conditions
- Sports injuries
- Posture-related issues

Scope of Practice and Collaboration: Chiropractors are primary healthcare providers in many countries and are licensed to diagnose and treat patients without a referral from a medical doctor. They often work collaboratively with other healthcare professionals, such as medical doctors, physical therapists, and massage therapists, to provide comprehensive care for their patients.

Efficacy and Safety: Research on the effectiveness of chiropractic care has shown positive outcomes for certain conditions, particularly musculoskeletal issues. Chiropractic treatment is generally considered safe when performed by a qualified and licensed chiropractor. However, like any medical intervention, it may not be suitable for everyone, and potential risks and benefits should be discussed with a healthcare provider before starting chiropractic care.

It's essential to choose a licensed and experienced chiropractor who has undergone proper training and education to ensure safe and effective treatment.

Understanding the concept of spinal alignment and nervous system

Spinal Alignment: Spinal alignment refers to the proper arrangement and positioning of the vertebral bones that make up the spine. The spine, also known as the vertebral column, serves as the central support structure of the body and is responsible for protecting the spinal cord while allowing flexibility and movement.

The spine consists of individual vertebral bones stacked on top of each other, separated by intervertebral discs that act as shock absorbers. There are three natural curves in the spine: the cervical (neck) curve, the thoracic (mid-back) curve, and the lumbar (lower back) curve. These curves help distribute the body's weight evenly, maintain balance, and absorb shock during movement.

Proper spinal alignment is essential for overall musculoskeletal health and nervous system function. When the spine is in alignment, the body is better able to maintain good posture, reduce stress on the joints, and allow smooth movement. On the other hand, spinal misalignments or subluxations can disrupt the body's balance and lead to various health issues.

Nervous System: The nervous system is a complex network of nerves, neurons, and other specialized cells that transmit electrical signals throughout the body. It plays a vital role in controlling and coordinating all bodily functions, including movement, sensation, perception, and organ function.

The nervous system can be divided into two main parts:

1. Central Nervous System (CNS): This includes the brain and spinal cord. The brain is responsible for processing information, making decisions, and controlling voluntary and involuntary actions. The spinal cord serves as a communication pathway between the brain and the rest of the body.
2. Peripheral Nervous System (PNS): This includes all the nerves that extend from the brain and spinal cord to other parts of the body. The PNS is further divided into the somatic nervous system, which controls voluntary movements and sensory perception, and the autonomic nervous system, which regulates involuntary functions like heart rate, digestion, and respiratory rate.

The nervous system relies on a continuous flow of information between the brain and various body parts. Sensory receptors in the skin, muscles, organs, and other tissues send signals to the brain, and the brain, in turn, sends messages back to the body to initiate appropriate responses.

Connection between Spinal Alignment and Nervous System: The spine plays a critical role in protecting the spinal cord, which is an extension of the brain and part of the central nervous system. The spinal cord transmits nerve impulses to and from the brain, allowing communication between the brain and the rest of the body.

When the spine is misaligned or subluxated, it can put pressure on the nerves that exit the spinal cord at various levels. This pressure can interfere with the transmission of nerve signals, leading to dysfunction, pain, and other health issues. Chiropractic care, which focuses on correcting spinal misalignments, aims to alleviate nerve interference and promote optimal nervous system function.

In summary, proper spinal alignment is essential for maintaining good posture, supporting movement, and reducing stress on the joints. It also plays a significant role in ensuring the proper functioning of the nervous system, which controls and coordinates all bodily processes. Chiropractic care, among other healthcare approaches, emphasizes the importance of spinal alignment in supporting overall health and well-being.

Techniques and adjustments
in chiropractic care

Chiropractic care utilizes various techniques and adjustments to address spinal misalignments or subluxations and promote proper spinal alignment. Each technique aims to restore joint function, reduce pain, and improve overall musculoskeletal health. Here are some common chiropractic techniques and adjustments:

1. Spinal Manipulation (Chiropractic Adjustment): This is the most well-known chiropractic technique and involves applying controlled force to specific areas of the spine to restore proper joint movement and alignment. Chiropractors use their hands or specialized instruments to deliver quick, controlled thrusts to the affected vertebrae. The goal is to reduce joint inflammation, improve mobility, and alleviate pain.
2. Flexion-Distraction Technique: This technique is commonly used to treat disc-related issues, such as herniated discs and sciatica. It involves gentle, rhythmic stretching of the spine while the patient is lying on a specialized table that moves in a controlled manner. Flexion-distraction helps decompress the discs, reduce pressure on the nerves, and improve spinal function.
3. Activator Method: The activator method uses a handheld, spring-loaded instrument called the Activator Adjusting Instrument to deliver precise, low-force adjustments to specific spinal segments. It is a gentle technique that is often used for patients who

prefer a less forceful adjustment or for individuals with certain health conditions that may require a more delicate approach.

4. Thompson Technique (Drop Table Technique): This technique involves the use of a special chiropractic table with drop sections. The table allows the chiropractor to apply a low-force adjustment to the spine by dropping specific sections of the table as the adjustment is performed. The dropping motion helps to facilitate the adjustment and minimize the force required.

5. Gonstead Technique: The Gonstead technique focuses on a thorough analysis of the spine to identify specific misalignments and areas of dysfunction. The chiropractor uses specific hand placements to deliver adjustments with precise and targeted force to the affected vertebrae.

6. Diversified Technique: The diversified technique is a more general, hands-on approach that involves a combination of manual adjustments and various chiropractic methods. The chiropractor uses their hands to apply quick thrusts to the spine to correct misalignments.

7. Cox Flexion-Distraction Technique: Similar to the flexion-distraction technique, the Cox technique involves gentle, repetitive stretching and mobilization of the spine using a specialized table. It is commonly used to treat conditions like disc herniations, spinal stenosis, and facet joint dysfunction.

8. Sacro-Occipital Technique (SOT): The SOT technique focuses on balancing the pelvis and the rest of the spine to optimize nervous system function. Chiropractors use blocks or wedges to support specific areas of the spine while applying gentle adjustments.

It's important to note that the choice of technique and adjustment used by a chiropractor will depend on the individual patient's condition, preferences, and overall health. Before undergoing any chiropractic treatment, it's essential to have a thorough evaluation and discussion with a qualified chiropractor to determine the most appropriate approach for your specific needs.

Conditions treated by chiropractors

Chiropractors primarily focus on diagnosing and treating conditions related to the musculoskeletal system, especially those involving the spine and nervous system. Some of the common conditions treated by chiropractors include:

1. Back Pain: Chiropractors are known for their expertise in treating various forms of back pain, including lower back pain, upper back pain, and chronic back conditions.
2. Neck Pain: Chiropractic care can be effective in alleviating neck pain caused by muscle strains, joint dysfunction, or other issues.
3. Headaches and Migraines: Chiropractic adjustments and spinal manipulation have been shown to provide relief for some individuals suffering from tension headaches and certain types of migraines.
4. Sciatica: Chiropractic care can help manage sciatica, a condition characterized by pain, numbness, or tingling that radiates along the sciatic nerve, which runs from the lower back down the legs.
5. Herniated Discs: Chiropractors may use various techniques to address herniated discs and reduce pressure on nerves causing pain and other symptoms.
6. Whiplash: Chiropractic care is commonly sought after motor vehicle accidents to address whiplash injuries, which can cause neck pain and stiffness.
7. Sports Injuries: Chiropractors work with athletes to treat and prevent sports-related injuries, such as sprains, strains, and joint problems.
8. Arthritis: Chiropractic care can help manage the pain

and stiffness associated with arthritis, especially in the spine and joints.

9. Scoliosis: While chiropractic care cannot correct scoliosis, it may help manage pain and discomfort associated with the condition.

10. Fibromyalgia: Chiropractic adjustments and other therapies may offer relief for some individuals with fibromyalgia by reducing muscle tension and promoting relaxation.

11. Repetitive Strain Injuries: Chiropractors can help address repetitive strain injuries, such as carpal tunnel syndrome and tennis elbow, often associated with work-related activities.

12. Pregnancy-related Pain: Chiropractors may offer gentle adjustments to help alleviate back pain and discomfort experienced during pregnancy.

It's important to note that chiropractors may also work in collaboration with other healthcare professionals to provide comprehensive care for patients. While chiropractic care is beneficial for many musculoskeletal conditions, it is essential to have a proper evaluation and diagnosis from a qualified healthcare provider to determine the most appropriate treatment approach for each individual's specific needs.

Integrating chiropractic with other holistic approaches

Integrating chiropractic care with other holistic approaches can provide a comprehensive and patient-centered approach to health and wellness. Holistic healthcare focuses on treating the whole person, considering physical, mental, emotional, and social factors that contribute to overall well-being. Here are some ways chiropractic care can be integrated with other holistic approaches:

1. Acupuncture: Chiropractic adjustments can be combined with acupuncture, an ancient Chinese healing practice that involves inserting thin needles into specific points on the body to stimulate energy flow and promote healing. The combination of chiropractic and acupuncture can address both musculoskeletal issues and imbalances in the body's energy system.

2. Massage Therapy: Chiropractic care can be complemented with massage therapy, which involves hands-on manipulation of muscles and soft tissues. Massage can help relax tense muscles, improve circulation, and enhance the effects of chiropractic adjustments.

3. Nutrition Counseling: Chiropractors may provide nutritional guidance to support overall health and address specific conditions. Proper nutrition plays a vital role in maintaining musculoskeletal health and supporting the body's natural healing processes.

4. Mind-Body Practices: Integrating chiropractic with mind-body practices such as yoga, meditation, or

mindfulness techniques can help manage stress, improve posture, and enhance the mind-body connection for overall well-being.

5. Herbal Medicine and Supplements: Chiropractors trained in herbal medicine may recommend specific herbs or supplements to complement chiropractic care and support the body's healing process.

6. Homeopathy: Homeopathic remedies, which use highly diluted substances to stimulate the body's healing response, can be integrated with chiropractic care to address specific health concerns.

7. Exercise and Physical Therapy: Chiropractors may collaborate with physical therapists to develop personalized exercise programs that support chiropractic treatments and help patients improve strength, flexibility, and mobility.

8. Holistic Lifestyle Coaching: Chiropractors may offer coaching on lifestyle factors such as sleep, stress management, and ergonomics to promote overall health and prevent future musculoskeletal issues.

9. Functional Medicine: Chiropractors trained in functional medicine may use diagnostic testing and personalized treatment plans to address the root causes of health issues and provide a more holistic approach to care.

10. Energy Healing: Integrating chiropractic with energy healing modalities such as Reiki or Healing Touch can enhance the body's natural healing abilities and promote balance and well-being.

It's essential for patients to communicate openly with their healthcare providers about their preferences and goals for treatment. A collaborative and integrative approach allows for a more comprehensive understanding of the individual's health and supports a multi-faceted treatment plan to promote optimal health and wellness.

Diet Therapy

Diet therapy, also known as medical nutrition therapy, is a specialized branch of healthcare that uses nutrition science to treat and manage various medical conditions. It involves the therapeutic use of specific diets and nutritional interventions to promote health, prevent disease, and manage the symptoms of existing health conditions. Diet therapy is typically prescribed and supervised by registered dietitians or healthcare professionals with expertise in nutrition.

Key principles of diet therapy include:

1. Individualized Approach: Diet therapy takes into account individual health needs, medical history, lifestyle, and personal preferences to develop personalized nutrition plans.
2. Evidence-Based Practice: Diet therapy is based on scientific evidence and clinical research, ensuring that the prescribed diets and interventions are effective and safe.
3. Disease Management: Diet therapy is commonly used to manage chronic diseases such as diabetes, cardiovascular disease, obesity, gastrointestinal disorders, and kidney disease.
4. Nutrient Balance: The goal of diet therapy is to achieve a balance of essential nutrients (carbohydrates, proteins, fats, vitamins, and minerals) to support optimal health and wellness.
5. Nutritional Education: Patients receive education and counseling about proper nutrition, portion control, label reading, and making healthy food choices.

6. Monitoring and Evaluation: Progress is regularly assessed, and nutrition plans may be adjusted based on changes in health status or treatment outcomes.

Conditions commonly managed with diet therapy include:

1. Diabetes: Dietary interventions play a crucial role in blood glucose control for individuals with diabetes.
2. Cardiovascular Disease: A heart-healthy diet can help manage high blood pressure, cholesterol levels, and reduce the risk of heart disease.
3. Gastrointestinal Disorders: Specific diets may be prescribed to manage conditions such as irritable bowel syndrome (IBS), celiac disease, and inflammatory bowel disease (IBD).
4. Obesity: Diet therapy can aid in weight management through personalized meal planning and behavior modification.
5. Renal Disease: Patients with kidney disease may require specific dietary restrictions to manage their condition.
6. Food Allergies and Intolerances: Diet therapy involves identifying and avoiding specific food triggers to manage allergic reactions or intolerances.
7. Malnutrition: Diet therapy can help address nutritional deficiencies and support recovery in individuals with malnutrition.

Diet therapy is an essential component of comprehensive healthcare and works in conjunction with medical treatments, medications, and lifestyle modifications to promote overall health and well-being. It emphasizes the importance of using food as medicine and harnessing the power of nutrition to enhance the body's natural healing abilities.

Role of diet in promoting health and preventing diseases

The role of diet in promoting health and preventing diseases is paramount. Nutrition plays a fundamental role in maintaining overall well-being and is a significant factor in reducing the risk of various chronic diseases. A balanced and nutritious diet provides essential nutrients that support bodily functions, boost the immune system, and help the body resist illnesses. Here are some key aspects of the role of diet in health promotion and disease prevention:

1. Nutrient Intake: A well-balanced diet provides essential nutrients such as carbohydrates, proteins, fats, vitamins, and minerals, which are necessary for the proper functioning of the body's organs and systems.
2. Weight Management: A healthy diet, combined with regular physical activity, helps maintain a healthy weight, reducing the risk of obesity and related health issues such as type 2 diabetes, heart disease, and certain cancers.
3. Heart Health: A diet rich in fruits, vegetables, whole grains, and lean proteins can help lower blood pressure, cholesterol levels, and the risk of heart disease and stroke.
4. Diabetes Prevention and Management: A balanced diet that regulates blood sugar levels can help prevent type 2 diabetes or manage the condition for those already diagnosed.
5. Digestive Health: Fiber-rich foods, such as fruits,

vegetables, and whole grains, promote healthy digestion and prevent constipation.

6. Bone Health: Adequate intake of calcium and vitamin D through the diet helps build and maintain strong bones, reducing the risk of osteoporosis.

7. Cancer Prevention: Certain foods, such as fruits, vegetables, and foods rich in antioxidants, may reduce the risk of developing certain types of cancer.

8. Mental Health: Nutrient-dense foods can positively influence mood and cognitive function, promoting better mental health.

9. Immune System Support: Proper nutrition supports a robust immune system, helping the body defend against infections and illnesses.

10. Energy and Vitality: A nutritious diet provides the energy needed for daily activities and helps maintain overall vitality and well-being.

To promote health and prevent diseases through diet:

- Emphasize a variety of fruits and vegetables, whole grains, lean proteins, and healthy fats in your meals.
- Limit the intake of processed and sugary foods, as well as excessive sodium and saturated fats.
- Stay hydrated by drinking plenty of water throughout the day.
- Practice portion control to prevent overeating and maintain a healthy weight.
- Engage in regular physical activity to complement a balanced diet and further promote health.

It is essential to work with healthcare professionals, such as registered dietitians or nutritionists, to develop personalized dietary plans that meet individual needs and health goals. By adopting a healthful and balanced diet, individuals can take proactive steps towards optimizing their health and reducing the risk of chronic diseases.

The impact of different food groups on the body

Different food groups have varying impacts on the body due to their unique nutrient composition. Each food group provides essential nutrients that serve specific functions in the body. Understanding the impact of different food groups can help individuals make informed and balanced dietary choices. Here are the primary food groups and their impacts on the body:

1. Fruits and Vegetables:
    - Provide vitamins, minerals, and antioxidants that support immune function and overall health.
    - High fiber content aids in digestion and promotes heart health.
    - Antioxidants help protect the body from oxidative stress and cellular damage.
2. Grains (Carbohydrates):
    - Serve as the body's primary source of energy.
    - Whole grains, such as brown rice and whole wheat, are rich in fiber, promoting digestive health and aiding in weight management.
3. Protein-Rich Foods (Meat, Fish, Legumes, Nuts, Seeds, Dairy, etc.):
    - Provide essential amino acids, which are building blocks for body tissues, enzymes, and hormones.
    - Play a critical role in muscle repair, growth, and maintenance.

- Support immune function and other essential bodily functions.

4. Dairy and Dairy Alternatives:
   - Rich sources of calcium and vitamin D, crucial for bone health and development.
   - Provide protein and other essential nutrients for overall health.

5. Fats and Oils:
   - Essential for energy storage and the absorption of fat-soluble vitamins (A, D, E, and K).
   - Omega-3 and Omega-6 fatty acids are vital for brain health and reducing inflammation.
   - Healthy fats, such as monounsaturated and polyunsaturated fats, support heart health.

6. Sugars and Sweets:
   - Provide quick energy but lack essential nutrients.
   - Excessive consumption can lead to weight gain, tooth decay, and an increased risk of chronic diseases when consumed in excess.

7. Processed and Packaged Foods:
   - Often high in sodium, added sugars, and unhealthy fats.
   - May lack essential nutrients found in whole foods.
   - Overconsumption can contribute to health issues, including obesity and heart disease.

A balanced diet that incorporates a variety of foods from different food groups is crucial for maintaining optimal health and well-being. Consuming a diverse array of nutrient-dense foods ensures that the body receives the necessary vitamins, minerals, and other nutrients for its proper functioning. It is essential to limit the intake of processed and unhealthy foods while focusing on whole, nutrient-rich options to support overall health and reduce the risk of chronic diseases. Remember that individual dietary needs vary based on age, activity level, and specific health conditions, so consulting with a healthcare professional or registered dietitian can provide personalized guidance.

Specific diets for various health conditions

There are several specific diets that have been studied and designed to address various health conditions. It's important to note that while some diets may show promising results for certain conditions, individual responses to diets can vary, and it's essential to consult with a healthcare professional or registered dietitian before making significant dietary changes. Here are some examples of specific diets for various health conditions:

1. Mediterranean Diet:
   - Recommended for: Heart health, weight management, and overall well-being.
   - Features: Rich in fruits, vegetables, whole grains, healthy fats (olive oil, nuts, seeds), moderate amounts of fish, poultry, and dairy, and limited red meat and processed foods.
2. DASH Diet (Dietary Approaches to Stop Hypertension):
   - Recommended for: Hypertension (high blood pressure) and cardiovascular health.
   - Features: Emphasizes fruits, vegetables, whole grains, lean proteins, and low-fat dairy while reducing sodium intake.
3. Ketogenic Diet:
   - Recommended for: Epilepsy (especially in children) and potential benefits in weight management and type 2 diabetes.
   - Features: High fat, very low carbohydrate, and moderate protein intake to induce a state of ketosis, where the body uses ketones for energy instead of glucose.

4. Gluten-Free Diet:
   - Recommended for: Celiac disease and gluten sensitivity.
   - Features: Eliminates all sources of gluten, a protein found in wheat, barley, and rye, to avoid triggering immune responses.
5. Low FODMAP Diet:
   - Recommended for: Irritable bowel syndrome (IBS) and digestive issues.
   - Features: Reduces fermentable carbohydrates (FODMAPs) that can cause gas, bloating, and abdominal pain.
6. Plant-Based Diet (Vegan or Vegetarian):
   - Recommended for: Overall health, weight management, and reducing the risk of certain chronic diseases.
   - Features: Focuses on plant-based foods, such as fruits, vegetables, whole grains, legumes, nuts, and seeds, while excluding or limiting animal products.
7. Anti-Inflammatory Diet:
   - Recommended for: Reducing chronic inflammation associated with certain health conditions.
   - Features: Emphasizes anti-inflammatory foods like fruits, vegetables, fatty fish, nuts, and seeds, while limiting processed foods, refined sugars, and unhealthy fats.
8. Specific Carbohydrate Diet (SCD):
   - Recommended for: Inflammatory bowel disease (IBD) and other digestive disorders.
   - Features: Eliminates complex carbohydrates and certain sugars to reduce inflammation and improve digestion.
9. Renal Diet:
   - Recommended for: Chronic kidney disease

(CKD).

- Features: Adjusts protein, phosphorus, potassium, and sodium intake to support kidney function and manage electrolyte imbalances.

These are just a few examples of specific diets for certain health conditions. Other diets, such as the GAPS diet for gut health, the Paleo diet for ancestral eating, and the MIND diet for brain health, are also worth mentioning. Always consult with a healthcare professional or registered dietitian to determine the most appropriate diet based on individual health needs, medical history, and lifestyle. They can help tailor a diet plan that best supports overall health and addresses specific health conditions.

Incorporating nutrition into holistic treatment plans

Incorporating nutrition into holistic treatment plans is a fundamental aspect of promoting overall health and well-being. Nutrition plays a vital role in supporting the body's natural healing processes and can complement other holistic therapies effectively. Here are some key steps to integrate nutrition into holistic treatment plans:

1. Comprehensive Assessment: Conduct a thorough assessment of the individual's health status, including medical history, current health conditions, lifestyle factors, dietary habits, and nutritional deficiencies, if any. This assessment helps create personalized nutrition plans tailored to the individual's unique needs.

2. Nutritional Counseling: Provide individualized nutritional counseling to educate and empower the individual on making informed food choices. A registered dietitian or nutritionist can guide them on selecting nutrient-dense foods, portion control, and addressing specific health concerns through dietary modifications.

3. Whole Foods Emphasis: Encourage the consumption of whole, unprocessed foods that are rich in vitamins, minerals, and other essential nutrients. Promote a balanced diet that includes a variety of fruits, vegetables, whole grains, lean proteins, and healthy fats.

4. Addressing Food Sensitivities: Identify and address any food sensitivities or allergies that may contribute

to health issues or exacerbate existing conditions. Eliminating or reducing trigger foods can lead to symptom improvement and overall well-being.

5. Supplements and Herbal Medicine: Integrate supplements or herbal medicine when appropriate to support specific health needs. However, it's essential to use supplements under the guidance of a healthcare professional to avoid potential interactions or adverse effects.

6. Mindful Eating: Encourage mindful eating practices, such as eating slowly, savoring food, and paying attention to hunger and fullness cues. Mindful eating promotes better digestion and helps individuals develop a positive relationship with food.

7. Hydration: Emphasize the importance of staying hydrated by consuming an adequate amount of water daily. Hydration is essential for proper body function and can support detoxification processes.

8. Collaborative Care: Work collaboratively with other healthcare practitioners involved in the individual's care, such as naturopaths, acupuncturists, chiropractors, and mental health professionals. Integrated care ensures that all aspects of the individual's health are addressed comprehensively.

9. Ongoing Monitoring and Adjustments: Continuously monitor the individual's progress and make necessary adjustments to the nutrition plan as needed. Regular follow-ups allow for modifications and improvements to enhance treatment outcomes.

10. Education and Empowerment: Educate individuals about the role of nutrition in their healing journey and how they can actively participate in their own well-being through proper nutrition and lifestyle choices.

Integrating nutrition into holistic treatment plans can enhance the effectiveness of other holistic therapies and provide a holistic approach to health and healing. It empowers individuals to take charge of their health and promotes optimal physical, mental, and emotional well-being. Always ensure that nutrition recommendations align with the individual's specific health needs and goals.

Holistic Medicine

Holistic medicine, also known as integrative or complementary medicine, is an approach to healthcare that considers the whole person – body, mind, spirit, and emotions – in the context of their environment. It goes beyond just treating symptoms and aims to address the root causes of health issues. The philosophy of holistic medicine is based on the belief that all aspects of a person's life are interconnected and influence their overall well-being.

Key Principles of Holistic Medicine:

1. Individualization: Holistic medicine recognizes that each person is unique and requires personalized care. Treatments and interventions are tailored to the individual's specific needs and health goals.
2. Integration: Holistic medicine seeks to integrate conventional medical practices with complementary therapies, such as acupuncture, chiropractic care, nutrition, herbal medicine, and mind-body techniques, to provide comprehensive care.
3. Prevention: Emphasizing preventive measures is a core principle of holistic medicine. Practitioners focus on promoting healthy lifestyle habits and empowering individuals to take an active role in maintaining their health.
4. Healing Partnership: The practitioner-patient relationship is viewed as a partnership, where both parties collaborate to achieve the best possible health outcomes. Holistic practitioners often spend more time with their patients, listening to their concerns and understanding the broader context of their lives.

5. Mind-Body-Spirit Connection: Holistic medicine recognizes the interconnectedness of physical, emotional, mental, and spiritual aspects of health. Emotional and spiritual well-being are considered essential components of overall health.
6. Natural Approaches: Holistic medicine emphasizes the use of natural therapies, such as herbal medicine, nutrition, and lifestyle modifications, to support the body's innate healing abilities.
7. Balance and Harmony: Holistic medicine seeks to restore balance and harmony within the body and mind. Imbalances are considered the root causes of illness, and treatment aims to address these imbalances.

Common Holistic Therapies and Modalities:

1. Acupuncture: Involves the insertion of thin needles into specific points on the body to stimulate energy flow and restore balance.
2. Chiropractic Care: Focuses on spinal adjustments and manipulations to alleviate pain and improve nervous system function.
3. Herbal Medicine: Uses plant-based remedies to support healing and address various health conditions.
4. Nutrition and Diet Therapy: Utilizes specific dietary approaches to support health and treat various health issues.
5. Mind-Body Techniques: Includes practices like meditation, yoga, mindfulness, and relaxation techniques to promote emotional and mental well-being.
6. Massage Therapy: Involves the manipulation of soft tissues to improve circulation, reduce muscle tension, and promote relaxation.
7. Energy Healing: Includes modalities like Reiki and healing touch, which aim to balance the body's energy

and promote healing.

Holistic medicine does not reject conventional medicine but rather seeks to complement and enhance it. It encourages a multidisciplinary approach to healthcare and recognizes the value of different healing modalities. As with any approach to healthcare, it is essential to work with qualified and experienced practitioners who can provide safe and effective treatments tailored to individual needs.

Holistic approach to healthcare and wellness

A holistic approach to healthcare and wellness considers the entire person – mind, body, spirit, and emotions – and recognizes the interconnectedness of all aspects of health. It goes beyond just treating symptoms and addresses the underlying root causes of health issues. The goal of a holistic approach is to promote overall well-being, prevent illness, and support the body's natural healing processes.

Key Elements of a Holistic Approach to Healthcare and Wellness:

1. Personalized Care: Each person is viewed as a unique individual with specific needs and health goals. Treatment plans are tailored to the individual, considering their medical history, lifestyle, preferences, and beliefs.
2. Integrative Therapies: Holistic healthcare often combines conventional medical practices with complementary and alternative therapies, such as acupuncture, chiropractic care, nutrition, herbal medicine, mindfulness, yoga, and meditation.
3. Prevention and Education: Holistic practitioners emphasize preventive measures and educate individuals about healthy lifestyle habits, nutrition, stress management, and self-care practices to maintain optimal health.
4. Mind-Body-Spirit Connection: A holistic approach recognizes the importance of emotional, mental, and spiritual well-being in overall health. Practices that promote relaxation, mindfulness, and emotional balance are integrated into treatment plans.

5. Natural and Non-Invasive Therapies: Holistic healthcare utilizes natural approaches to support the body's healing processes and minimize the use of invasive procedures and medications when possible.
6. Balance and Harmony: The focus is on restoring balance and harmony within the body, as imbalances are considered the underlying causes of illness.
7. Patient-Centered Care: Holistic practitioners take the time to listen to their patients, understand their concerns, and involve them in the decision-making process regarding their health.
8. Lifestyle Modifications: Emphasis is placed on adopting healthy lifestyle habits, including a balanced diet, regular exercise, adequate sleep, and stress reduction.
9. Long-Term Health: The goal of holistic healthcare is not only to treat acute conditions but also to support long-term health and wellness.

Benefits of a Holistic Approach to Healthcare and Wellness:

- Improved overall health and well-being
- Prevention of chronic diseases
- Enhanced self-awareness and empowerment in managing health
- Reduced reliance on medications and invasive procedures
- Increased focus on root causes of health issues
- Better management of chronic conditions
- Promotion of emotional and mental well-being
- Greater sense of balance and harmony in life

It's essential to work with qualified and experienced holistic healthcare practitioners who can provide evidence-based and safe treatments. A holistic approach can be integrated with conventional medicine to create a comprehensive healthcare plan that meets the individual's unique needs and supports their journey toward optimal health and wellness.

Integrating mind, body, and spirit in treatment

Integrating mind, body, and spirit in treatment is a key principle of holistic healthcare, aiming to address the interconnectedness of these aspects in promoting overall well-being. This approach recognizes that a person's mental, emotional, physical, and spiritual health are interconnected and influence each other. By considering and addressing all these dimensions, healthcare providers can offer more comprehensive and effective treatments.

1. Mind: The mental aspect of health includes thoughts, beliefs, emotions, and cognitive processes. Integrating the mind in treatment involves addressing psychological factors, such as stress, anxiety, depression, and trauma. Mindfulness practices, meditation, cognitive-behavioral therapy (CBT), and other psychotherapeutic techniques can be employed to support mental well-being.

2. Body: The physical aspect of health refers to the body's physiological functions and structures. Integrating the body in treatment involves addressing physical health conditions, providing nutrition and exercise recommendations, and using body-based therapies like massage, chiropractic adjustments, and acupuncture to promote healing and relaxation.

3. Spirit: The spiritual aspect of health encompasses an individual's sense of purpose, meaning, and connection to something greater than oneself. Integrating the spirit in treatment involves exploring a person's values,

beliefs, and sense of purpose. Practices like meditation, yoga, prayer, and engaging in nature can support spiritual well-being.

Integrative and Holistic Treatments:

1. Mind-Body Techniques: Mind-body therapies, such as yoga, meditation, guided imagery, and biofeedback, are used to foster a connection between mental and physical well-being. These practices can reduce stress, improve mood, and enhance overall health.
2. Nutritional Counseling: Nutrition plays a vital role in overall health. Integrative healthcare providers offer personalized dietary recommendations to support physical and mental well-being.
3. Exercise and Physical Activity: Regular physical activity can have numerous physical and mental health benefits. Integrative practitioners may recommend specific exercise regimens tailored to an individual's needs and preferences.
4. Energy Healing: Modalities like Reiki, healing touch, and acupuncture are based on the concept of energy flow in the body. These practices aim to restore balance and promote healing by addressing energetic imbalances.
5. Mindfulness-Based Therapies: Mindfulness-based therapies, such as Mindfulness-Based Stress Reduction (MBSR) and Mindfulness-Based Cognitive Therapy (MBCT), integrate mindfulness practices with traditional psychotherapy to enhance mental well-being.
6. Art Therapy: Art therapy uses creative expression as a means of exploring emotions, reducing stress, and promoting self-awareness.

Integrating mind, body, and spirit in treatment allows healthcare providers to address health issues from a more comprehensive perspective. It empowers individuals to actively participate in their healing journey and promotes a deeper understanding of the factors influencing their well-being. By considering the interconnected nature of these aspects, holistic healthcare can support overall health and healing on multiple levels.

The role of complementary therapies in holistic medicine

Complementary therapies play a crucial role in holistic medicine by providing additional approaches and treatments that support the overall well-being of individuals. These therapies work alongside conventional medical practices to address the physical, mental, emotional, and spiritual aspects of health. The integration of complementary therapies in holistic medicine aims to enhance the body's natural healing mechanisms and promote a sense of balance and harmony within the individual.

Key Roles of Complementary Therapies in Holistic Medicine:

1. Addressing the Whole Person: Complementary therapies take into account the interconnected nature of an individual's physical, emotional, mental, and spiritual health. They recognize that addressing one aspect of health can have positive effects on other aspects.

2. Supporting Conventional Treatments: Complementary therapies can enhance the effectiveness of conventional medical treatments by reducing side effects, improving treatment outcomes, and supporting the body's ability to heal.

3. Empowering Individuals: Complementary therapies often empower individuals to take an active role in their healing process. Practices like mindfulness, meditation, and self-care techniques enable individuals to manage stress and improve their overall well-being.

4. Reducing Stress and Anxiety: Many complementary therapies, such as acupuncture, massage, and meditation, are effective in reducing stress and anxiety, which can contribute to improved physical and mental health.
5. Enhancing Pain Management: Complementary therapies like acupuncture, chiropractic care, and massage can be effective in managing pain and promoting relaxation.
6. Promoting Prevention and Wellness: Complementary therapies often focus on prevention and promoting a healthy lifestyle, which can help prevent the onset of chronic diseases and promote long-term wellness.

Examples of Complementary Therapies in Holistic Medicine:

1. Acupuncture: Based on traditional Chinese medicine, acupuncture involves inserting thin needles into specific points on the body to balance the flow of energy (Qi) and promote healing.
2. Chiropractic Care: Chiropractors use manual adjustments to align the spine and promote the proper functioning of the nervous system, which can improve overall health.
3. Herbal Medicine: The use of herbs and plant-based remedies to support the body's natural healing processes and address specific health concerns.
4. Mindfulness and Meditation: Practices that promote awareness of the present moment and a sense of inner calm, reducing stress and improving mental well-being.
5. Massage Therapy: Manipulation of soft tissues to reduce muscle tension, improve circulation, and promote relaxation.
6. Yoga: A mind-body practice that combines physical postures, breathwork, and meditation to improve flexibility, strength, and overall well-being.

7. Reiki: A form of energy healing that aims to balance and restore the flow of energy in the body, promoting relaxation and healing.

Integrating complementary therapies into holistic medicine provides a more comprehensive and patient-centered approach to healthcare. It allows individuals to access a wide range of treatment options that can be tailored to their unique needs and preferences. Additionally, by addressing the whole person, complementary therapies contribute to a holistic approach to healing and wellness. It's essential to work with qualified and experienced practitioners who can provide evidence-based and safe complementary therapies as part of a comprehensive healthcare plan.

Holistic healing techniques and practices

Holistic healing techniques and practices focus on addressing the whole person, including physical, mental, emotional, and spiritual aspects of health. These practices aim to promote balance, harmony, and well-being by considering the interconnectedness of the individual and their environment. Here are some common holistic healing techniques and practices:

1. Mindfulness and Meditation: Mindfulness practices involve being fully present in the moment, observing thoughts and emotions without judgment. Meditation techniques can vary and may include focused attention, loving-kindness meditation, or body scan meditation.
2. Yoga: Yoga combines physical postures, breathwork, and meditation to promote flexibility, strength, and relaxation. It has both physical and mental health benefits and can reduce stress and anxiety.
3. Acupuncture: Based on traditional Chinese medicine, acupuncture involves inserting thin needles into specific points on the body to balance the flow of energy and promote healing.
4. Massage Therapy: Manipulation of soft tissues to relieve muscle tension, improve circulation, and promote relaxation. Different types of massage, such as Swedish massage, deep tissue massage, and aromatherapy massage, can address various needs.
5. Herbal Medicine: The use of plant-based remedies, herbs, and botanicals to support the body's natural healing processes and address specific health concerns.
6. Chiropractic Care: Chiropractors use manual

adjustments to align the spine and promote proper nervous system functioning, which can improve overall health.

7. Reiki and Energy Healing: Energy healing modalities aim to balance and restore the flow of energy in the body, promoting relaxation and healing.

8. Nutrition and Dietary Counseling: A focus on wholesome and balanced nutrition to support overall health and well-being. Nutritional counseling may involve personalized dietary recommendations and lifestyle changes.

9. Aromatherapy: The use of essential oils derived from plants to promote physical and emotional well-being. Essential oils can be used in aromatherapy diffusers, massage oils, or bath products.

10. Art Therapy: Using creative expression as a means of exploring emotions, reducing stress, and promoting self-awareness.

11. Hydrotherapy: The use of water in various forms, such as hot baths, saunas, or steam rooms, for therapeutic purposes, relaxation, and pain relief.

12. Music Therapy: Utilizing music to support emotional expression, reduce anxiety, and enhance overall well-being.

13. Breathwork: Breathing exercises and techniques to promote relaxation, reduce stress, and improve mental clarity.

14. Sound Healing: Using sound vibrations, such as singing bowls or chanting, to promote relaxation and a sense of harmony.

15. Forest Bathing (Shinrin-Yoku): Spending time in nature to reduce stress, improve mood, and enhance overall well-being.

It's important to note that while holistic healing techniques can be beneficial for many individuals, they are not meant to replace conventional medical treatments for serious health conditions. If you are considering incorporating holistic healing practices into your wellness routine, it is advisable to consult with qualified practitioners and healthcare professionals to ensure safe and appropriate integration with other aspects of your healthcare.

Hypnotherapy

Hypnotherapy is a therapeutic technique that uses hypnosis to promote relaxation, focus, and concentration. During a hypnotherapy session, a trained therapist guides the individual into a state of deep relaxation, known as a hypnotic trance. In this trance-like state, the individual becomes more open to suggestions and is more receptive to positive changes in thoughts, feelings, and behaviors.

Key Aspects of Hypnotherapy:

1. Hypnotic Induction: The process of guiding the individual into a state of deep relaxation and heightened focus, also known as the hypnotic trance. This is typically achieved through verbal guidance and relaxation techniques.
2. Suggestion: While in the hypnotic trance, the therapist may provide positive and beneficial suggestions to the individual's subconscious mind. These suggestions are intended to help the individual overcome challenges, change negative thought patterns, or promote desired behavioral changes.
3. Increased Awareness: In the hypnotic trance, individuals often experience heightened awareness and focus on their internal experiences and sensations.
4. Goal-Oriented Approach: Hypnotherapy is often used to address specific issues or goals, such as reducing anxiety, managing pain, overcoming phobias, improving sleep, enhancing self-confidence, or breaking unwanted habits.
5. Subconscious Influence: Hypnotherapy aims to work

with the subconscious mind, where beliefs, emotions, and automatic responses are thought to be stored. By accessing the subconscious, individuals can explore and modify thought patterns and behaviors.

6. Relaxation and Stress Reduction: The deep relaxation experienced during hypnotherapy sessions can help reduce stress and promote overall well-being.

Benefits of Hypnotherapy:

1. Stress and Anxiety Reduction: Hypnotherapy can help individuals manage stress, anxiety, and related symptoms by promoting relaxation and providing coping strategies.
2. Pain Management: Hypnotherapy can be effective in managing chronic pain and helping individuals cope with discomfort.
3. Behavioral Changes: Hypnotherapy can aid in breaking unwanted habits, such as smoking or overeating, by promoting positive behavioral changes.
4. Phobia and Fear Resolution: Hypnotherapy can be used to address and overcome specific phobias and fears.
5. Improved Sleep: Hypnotherapy may help improve sleep quality and address insomnia-related issues.
6. Enhanced Self-Confidence and Performance: Hypnotherapy can be used to boost self-esteem and enhance performance in various areas, such as public speaking or sports.

It's important to note that while hypnotherapy can be beneficial for many individuals, its effectiveness may vary from person to person. Additionally, hypnotherapy should always be conducted by a trained and certified hypnotherapist to ensure safety and ethical practices.

Hypnotherapy is considered a complementary therapy and is often used in conjunction with other forms of treatment.

Individuals interested in exploring hypnotherapy should discuss their options with a qualified healthcare provider or seek a licensed hypnotherapist who has experience in their specific area of interest or concern.

Understanding the power of the subconscious mind

The subconscious mind is a powerful aspect of our mental functioning that plays a significant role in shaping our thoughts, emotions, behaviors, and overall experiences. It operates below the level of conscious awareness and is responsible for storing a vast amount of information, beliefs, memories, and automatic responses. Understanding the power of the subconscious mind can provide valuable insights into how our minds work and how we can harness its potential for personal growth and positive change.

Key Aspects of the Subconscious Mind:

1. Storage of Information: The subconscious mind acts as a vast repository, storing all kinds of information, experiences, and memories, even those that we may not be consciously aware of.
2. Automatic Processes: Many of our daily actions and reactions are driven by the subconscious mind. It controls automatic processes like breathing, heart rate, and digestion, as well as ingrained habits and learned behaviors.
3. Emotional Responses: The subconscious mind strongly influences emotional responses. Past experiences and associations stored in the subconscious can trigger emotional reactions in the present.
4. Beliefs and Values: Our beliefs, values, and self-image are deeply rooted in the subconscious mind. These

beliefs can impact our perceptions of ourselves and the world, shaping our thoughts and actions.

5. Creative Problem-Solving: The subconscious mind is highly creative and can contribute to problem-solving and generating new ideas and insights.
6. Power of Suggestion: The subconscious mind is receptive to suggestion, especially in states of relaxation or trance. This aspect is often used in hypnotherapy and positive affirmations to bring about desired changes.

Harnessing the Power of the Subconscious Mind:

1. Visualization and Affirmations: Using positive visualization and affirmations can help reprogram the subconscious mind with empowering beliefs and goals.
2. Hypnotherapy: Hypnotherapy is a powerful tool to access and influence the subconscious mind. Through relaxation and suggestion, positive changes can be made at the subconscious level.
3. Meditation: Meditation allows us to quiet the conscious mind and access the deeper layers of the subconscious. It can promote self-awareness and facilitate positive transformation.
4. Mindfulness: Practicing mindfulness helps bring attention to the present moment and observe subconscious thoughts and patterns without judgment.
5. Repetition: Repeatedly exposing the subconscious mind to positive and constructive messages can gradually create new neural pathways and beliefs.
6. Emotional Release: Emotionally processing past traumas or negative experiences can release their hold on the subconscious and promote healing.

It is essential to remember that the subconscious mind does not distinguish between positive and negative thoughts or beliefs. Therefore, it is crucial to focus on fostering positive and constructive thinking to optimize the power of the subconscious mind for personal growth and well-being.

While the subconscious mind has great potential for positive change, it is also essential to recognize that it is just one aspect of the mind. Integrating the conscious and subconscious aspects of the mind can lead to a more balanced and harmonious life. Seeking professional guidance from therapists, coaches, or counselors experienced in working with the subconscious mind can be beneficial for those seeking to explore and utilize its potential.

Inducing hypnosis and guiding clients through therapy

Inducing hypnosis and guiding clients through therapy is a specialized skill performed by trained hypnotherapists. The process involves helping clients achieve a state of deep relaxation and focus, known as a hypnotic trance, where they become more receptive to positive suggestions and therapeutic interventions. Here is an overview of how hypnosis is induced and how clients are guided through therapy:

1. Preparing the Client: Before starting the hypnosis session, the hypnotherapist establishes rapport with the client and discusses their goals and concerns. It is essential to create a safe and trusting environment to ensure the client feels comfortable and at ease.

2. Inducing Hypnosis: Hypnosis can be induced using various techniques, such as progressive relaxation, guided imagery, or focused attention. The goal is to lead the client into a state of deep relaxation, where their conscious mind becomes less dominant, and their subconscious mind becomes more accessible.

3. Deepening the Trance: Once the client is in a relaxed state, the hypnotherapist may use further techniques to deepen the hypnotic trance. This can involve suggestions for increasing relaxation, visualizations, or counting down from a specific number.

4. Positive Suggestions: While the client is in the hypnotic trance, the hypnotherapist provides positive and beneficial suggestions related to the client's therapeutic

goals. These suggestions are tailored to address specific issues, such as reducing anxiety, boosting confidence, or breaking unwanted habits.

5. Therapeutic Interventions: In addition to positive suggestions, the hypnotherapist may use various therapeutic techniques during the trance to address the client's needs. These may include cognitive-behavioral strategies, visualization exercises, or regression therapy to explore past experiences.

6. Post-Hypnotic Suggestions: Towards the end of the session, the hypnotherapist may provide post-hypnotic suggestions, which are instructions given to the client's subconscious to continue the positive changes beyond the session.

7. Gradual Awakening: After completing the therapeutic work, the hypnotherapist guides the client back to full awareness and a state of wakefulness. Clients typically feel relaxed and refreshed after the session.

It is important to note that hypnosis is a cooperative process, and the client must be willing and open to the experience. Hypnotherapy is not mind control, and clients cannot be made to do anything against their will or values. The effectiveness of hypnotherapy varies from person to person, and results may not be immediate, requiring multiple sessions for lasting change.

Professional hypnotherapists undergo rigorous training and certification to ensure ethical and safe practices. If you are interested in exploring hypnotherapy for specific concerns or goals, seek a licensed and qualified hypnotherapist with experience in the areas you wish to address.

Applications of hypnotherapy in stress reduction, pain management, etc.

Hypnotherapy has a wide range of applications in various areas of health and well-being. Some of the key areas where hypnotherapy is used include:

1. Stress Reduction: Hypnotherapy can be effective in reducing stress and promoting relaxation. During hypnosis, clients can access a state of deep relaxation, which helps in calming the mind and reducing stress-related symptoms.
2. Pain Management: Hypnotherapy has been used to alleviate chronic pain, such as migraines, arthritis, and fibromyalgia. Hypnosis can help change the perception of pain and reduce its intensity.
3. Anxiety and Phobia Treatment: Hypnotherapy can assist individuals in managing anxiety and overcoming specific phobias. It helps in addressing the root causes of anxiety and creating a more positive response to triggers.
4. Smoking Cessation: Hypnotherapy is used to support individuals in quitting smoking by breaking the habit and reducing withdrawal symptoms.
5. Weight Management: Hypnotherapy can be part of weight management programs by addressing emotional eating, promoting healthier eating habits, and encouraging motivation for exercise.
6. Sleep Disorders: Hypnotherapy can aid in improving sleep patterns and overcoming insomnia by inducing

relaxation and promoting better sleep hygiene.

7. Confidence and Self-Esteem: Hypnotherapy can help boost self-confidence and self-esteem by working on underlying beliefs and promoting a more positive self-image.

8. Performance Enhancement: Hypnotherapy is used to enhance performance in various areas, including sports, public speaking, and academic exams.

9. Trauma and PTSD: Hypnotherapy can be a part of a comprehensive treatment plan for individuals dealing with trauma or post-traumatic stress disorder (PTSD).

10. Behavioral Changes: Hypnotherapy can address various unwanted behaviors, such as nail-biting, hair-pulling, and other habits.

11. Emotional Healing: Hypnotherapy can assist in emotional healing by helping individuals process past traumas and negative emotions.

12. Coping with Medical Procedures: Hypnotherapy is sometimes used to help individuals cope with medical procedures, such as dental work or surgery, by reducing anxiety and discomfort.

It is essential to remember that hypnotherapy is most effective when used as part of an integrated treatment plan tailored to the individual's specific needs and goals. It should be administered by a trained and licensed hypnotherapist who understands the client's concerns and provides personalized sessions.

Hypnotherapy is generally considered safe when practiced by qualified professionals. However, it may not be suitable for everyone, and individuals with certain mental health conditions or medical issues should consult with their healthcare provider before undergoing hypnotherapy.

Ethical considerations in hypnotherapy practice

Ethical considerations are essential in any therapeutic practice, including hypnotherapy. As hypnotherapy involves working with a person's subconscious mind and vulnerability, adhering to ethical guidelines ensures the safety, well-being, and confidentiality of the client. Some key ethical considerations in hypnotherapy practice include:

1. Informed Consent: Obtaining informed consent is critical before starting any hypnotherapy session. Clients should be fully aware of what hypnosis entails, the purpose of the session, potential benefits, and any risks involved. They should also be informed that they can terminate the session at any time.

2. Competence and Training: Hypnotherapists must have appropriate training, qualifications, and experience in the field. They should only practice within the scope of their training and competence, ensuring the well-being of the clients.

3. Confidentiality: Hypnotherapists must maintain strict confidentiality regarding all information disclosed by the client during sessions. Clients should be assured that their personal information will not be shared without their explicit permission, except in cases where mandated by law or when there is a risk of harm to self or others.

4. Respect and Non-Discrimination: Hypnotherapists should treat all clients with respect and dignity, regardless of their background, beliefs, or lifestyle. They should not discriminate based on race, ethnicity,

religion, gender, sexual orientation, or any other characteristic.

5. Beneficence and Non-Maleficence: Hypnotherapists have a duty to act in the best interest of their clients and avoid causing harm. They should prioritize the well-being and safety of the client at all times.

6. Boundaries and Dual Relationships: Hypnotherapists should maintain appropriate professional boundaries and avoid dual relationships that could impair objectivity or lead to conflicts of interest.

7. Cultural Competence: Hypnotherapists should be sensitive to cultural differences and be aware of how cultural factors may impact the therapeutic process.

8. Advertising and Marketing: Hypnotherapists should ensure that their advertising and marketing materials are truthful, accurate, and do not make unrealistic promises about the benefits of hypnotherapy.

9. Continuing Education: Hypnotherapists should engage in ongoing professional development and stay informed about new developments and research in the field.

10. Supervision and Consultation: Hypnotherapists should seek supervision or consultation when needed to ensure that they are providing effective and ethical care to their clients.

Adhering to ethical principles is essential to maintain the integrity and credibility of hypnotherapy as a therapeutic modality. It helps build trust between the hypnotherapist and the client, leading to more positive therapeutic outcomes. Hypnotherapists should also be aware of any legal and regulatory requirements in their region related to hypnotherapy practice.

Mind-Body Medicine (Psychoneuroimmunology)

Mind-body medicine, also known as psychoneuroimmunology (PNI), is an interdisciplinary field that explores the connection between the mind, body, and immune system. It investigates how thoughts, emotions, behaviors, and social factors influence physical health and well-being. The underlying principle of mind-body medicine is that the mind and body are interconnected and that psychological, emotional, and social factors can significantly impact physical health.

Key Concepts in Mind-Body Medicine:

1. Psychoneuroimmunology (PNI): PNI is the scientific study of the interactions between psychological processes, the nervous system, and the immune system. It examines how the mind and body communicate with each other through various pathways, including neural, hormonal, and immunological pathways.

2. Stress Response: The stress response is a central aspect of mind-body medicine. Chronic stress can negatively affect the immune system, making individuals more susceptible to illness and disease. Mind-body interventions aim to reduce stress and promote relaxation, which can enhance overall health.

3. Placebo and Nocebo Effects: The placebo effect refers to the improvement of symptoms or health outcomes due to the belief in a treatment, even if the treatment itself has no therapeutic value. Conversely, the nocebo effect

occurs when negative outcomes are experienced due to negative expectations or beliefs about a treatment or situation.

4. Mind-Body Techniques: Mind-body medicine incorporates a variety of techniques and practices to promote health and well-being. These techniques may include relaxation techniques (e.g., meditation, progressive muscle relaxation), biofeedback, guided imagery, mindfulness practices, and cognitive-behavioral therapies.

5. Emotional Health and Immunity: Emotions can have a significant impact on immune function. Positive emotions, such as joy, love, and gratitude, have been associated with enhanced immune responses, while negative emotions, such as stress, anxiety, and depression, can weaken the immune system.

6. Social Support: Strong social support networks have been linked to better health outcomes and improved immunity. Social connections can buffer the effects of stress and provide emotional support, which contributes to overall well-being.

Applications of Mind-Body Medicine:

Mind-body medicine is utilized in various healthcare settings and has been integrated into traditional medical practices. It is often used as a complementary approach to support conventional medical treatments. Mind-body interventions have been applied in the management of various conditions, including chronic pain, cardiovascular diseases, cancer, autoimmune disorders, and mental health conditions.

Benefits of Mind-Body Medicine:

- Reducing stress and anxiety
- Enhancing immune function
- Improving emotional well-being

- Promoting relaxation and sleep
- Supporting pain management
- Enhancing coping skills and resilience

It is important to note that mind-body medicine should not replace conventional medical treatments. Instead, it can be used in conjunction with standard medical care to optimize health and well-being. Before incorporating mind-body practices, individuals should consult with healthcare professionals to ensure safety and appropriateness for their specific health conditions.

The mind-body connection in health and disease

The mind-body connection refers to the intricate interplay between our mental and emotional states and our physical health. It highlights the profound influence that thoughts, emotions, beliefs, and behaviors can have on our overall well-being and the development or management of diseases. The mind and body are intricately linked, and changes in one can impact the other.

Key Aspects of the Mind-Body Connection:

1. Stress Response: When we encounter stressful situations or experience negative emotions, our body activates the "fight or flight" response, releasing stress hormones like cortisol and adrenaline. Chronic stress and negative emotions can weaken the immune system, making individuals more susceptible to illness and exacerbating existing health conditions.

2. Placebo and Nocebo Effects: The placebo effect occurs when a person experiences improvements in symptoms or health outcomes after receiving a treatment with no therapeutic value, solely due to their belief in the treatment's effectiveness. On the other hand, the nocebo effect occurs when negative outcomes are experienced due to negative expectations or beliefs about a treatment or situation.

3. Immune System: Emotional well-being can directly impact the functioning of the immune system. Positive emotions, such as happiness and optimism, have been

associated with enhanced immune responses, while negative emotions, such as depression and anxiety, can suppress immune function.

4. Mind-Body Interventions: Mind-body techniques, such as meditation, mindfulness, yoga, biofeedback, and guided imagery, can positively influence both mental and physical health. These practices promote relaxation, reduce stress, and enhance overall well-being.

5. Chronic Conditions: Psychological factors can influence the onset and progression of chronic diseases. For example, stress and emotional distress have been linked to cardiovascular diseases, autoimmune disorders, gastrointestinal issues, and other conditions.

6. Mind-Body Medicine: The field of mind-body medicine explores the connection between the mind, body, and health. It emphasizes the use of integrative and holistic approaches to support overall well-being and the treatment of illnesses.

The Importance of the Mind-Body Connection in Health and Disease:

Understanding the mind-body connection is crucial for healthcare professionals and individuals alike because it highlights the need to consider both psychological and physical aspects of health. By recognizing the impact of stress, emotions, and lifestyle on health, individuals can take proactive steps to improve their well-being.

Promoting a healthy mind-body connection can:

1. Improve overall health and well-being: By adopting positive coping strategies, managing stress, and fostering emotional resilience, individuals can enhance their physical and mental health.

2. Enhance disease management: Integrating mind-body techniques with medical treatments can improve

outcomes and quality of life for individuals managing chronic conditions.

3. Support preventive care: Addressing emotional and psychological factors can help prevent the development of certain health conditions and promote a proactive approach to health.

4. Optimize healing and recovery: A positive mindset and emotional support can aid the healing process and recovery from illnesses and medical procedures.

5. Encourage a holistic approach to healthcare: Recognizing the mind-body connection encourages a more comprehensive and integrated approach to healthcare that considers all aspects of a person's health.

In summary, the mind-body connection plays a significant role in health and disease. By recognizing and nurturing this connection, individuals can take an active role in promoting their well-being and optimizing their overall health. Healthcare professionals can incorporate mind-body approaches into their practice to support patients' physical and emotional health.

Techniques for managing stress and improving mental health

Managing stress and improving mental health are essential for maintaining overall well-being. Here are some effective techniques that can help:

1. Mindfulness Meditation: Practicing mindfulness involves being fully present in the moment without judgment. Mindfulness meditation can reduce stress, anxiety, and depressive symptoms while promoting a sense of calm and clarity.

2. Deep Breathing Exercises: Deep breathing exercises, such as diaphragmatic breathing, can activate the body's relaxation response, reducing stress and promoting relaxation.

3. Physical Exercise: Regular physical activity, such as walking, jogging, yoga, or dancing, releases endorphins, the body's natural mood elevators, which can help alleviate stress and improve mental health.

4. Social Support: Connecting with friends, family, or support groups can provide emotional support, reduce feelings of isolation, and improve mental well-being.

5. Time Management: Prioritizing tasks, setting realistic goals, and managing time efficiently can reduce stress and create a sense of accomplishment.

6. Healthy Eating: A balanced diet with plenty of fruits, vegetables, whole grains, and lean proteins supports mental health and provides essential nutrients for brain function.

7. **Adequate Sleep:** Getting enough quality sleep is crucial for mental health and can help reduce stress and improve cognitive function.

8. **Limiting Stimulants:** Reducing or avoiding caffeine, alcohol, and other stimulants can help manage anxiety and improve sleep quality.

9. **Creative Expression:** Engaging in creative activities such as writing, drawing, painting, or playing music can be therapeutic and help process emotions.

10. **Practicing Gratitude:** Keeping a gratitude journal or regularly reflecting on things you are thankful for can shift focus away from stress and promote a positive outlook.

11. **Cognitive Behavioral Therapy (CBT):** CBT is a widely used form of therapy that helps individuals identify and change negative thought patterns and behaviors.

12. **Seek Professional Help:** If stress or mental health issues become overwhelming, seeking help from a mental health professional, such as a psychologist or counselor, can provide guidance and support.

13. **Limiting Media Exposure:** Reducing exposure to negative news or social media can help decrease stress and anxiety.

14. **Engaging in Relaxation Techniques:** Relaxation techniques such as progressive muscle relaxation, guided imagery, or aromatherapy can promote relaxation and reduce stress.

15. **Nature and Outdoor Activities:** Spending time in nature or engaging in outdoor activities can have a positive impact on mental health and reduce stress.

Remember that everyone is unique, and what works for one person may not work for another. It's essential to find strategies that resonate with you and incorporate them into your daily routine to manage stress and support mental health effectively. If stress or mental health challenges persist, seeking professional

guidance is always recommended.

Psychoneuroimmunology and its impact on the immune system

Psychoneuroimmunology (PNI) is a multidisciplinary field that examines the interactions between the nervous, endocrine, and immune systems. It explores how psychological factors, such as stress, emotions, and mental state, influence the immune system's functioning and, consequently, overall health.

The immune system is a complex network of cells, tissues, and organs that work together to defend the body against pathogens (e.g., bacteria, viruses) and other foreign substances. It also plays a crucial role in identifying and eliminating abnormal or damaged cells, such as cancer cells. The immune system's proper functioning is essential for maintaining optimal health and preventing illnesses.

PNI research has demonstrated that psychological stress can have a significant impact on the immune system. Chronic stress, in particular, has been associated with negative changes in immune function, including:

1. Inflammation: Chronic stress can lead to increased production of pro-inflammatory cytokines, which contribute to inflammation in the body. This inflammation, if prolonged, may contribute to various health conditions, such as cardiovascular disease, autoimmune disorders, and certain mental health issues.

2. Immune Suppression: Chronic stress can suppress the immune system's activity, making the body more

vulnerable to infections and impairing the body's ability to fight off illnesses.

3. Delayed Wound Healing: Stress can delay wound healing by affecting the immune response required for tissue repair.
4. Alterations in Immune Cells: Stress can lead to changes in the distribution and function of immune cells, potentially compromising the body's ability to mount an effective immune response.

Conversely, positive emotions, social support, and relaxation techniques have been associated with positive effects on the immune system. For example:

1. Positive emotions and social connections can stimulate the release of endorphins and oxytocin, which can enhance immune function.
2. Mind-body practices like meditation and yoga have been shown to reduce stress and inflammation while promoting immune system health.
3. Engaging in regular physical activity can support immune function and overall well-being.

Overall, psychoneuroimmunology highlights the interconnectedness of psychological and physiological processes and emphasizes the importance of maintaining a balance between mental and physical health. Managing stress, promoting positive emotions, and adopting healthy lifestyle habits are essential for supporting the immune system and overall well-being. However, it's crucial to remember that the immune system is complex, and various factors influence its function, including genetics, diet, and environmental exposures. As such, a holistic approach to health that considers the interplay between mind, body, and environment is vital for maintaining a robust immune system and overall health.

Mindfulness and meditation practices

Mindfulness and meditation practices are ancient techniques that promote awareness, presence, and focus on the present moment. They have been adopted in various cultures and are now widely recognized and used in modern settings to improve mental and emotional well-being. These practices can be valuable tools for reducing stress, enhancing self-awareness, managing emotions, and fostering overall mental clarity and calmness.

1. Mindfulness: Mindfulness involves paying non-judgmental attention to the present moment, accepting thoughts and feelings as they arise without reacting to them. It involves being fully present in the here and now, observing thoughts and sensations without getting entangled in them. Mindfulness practices can include simple activities like mindful breathing, eating, or walking, as well as formal meditation techniques.

2. Meditation: Meditation refers to a wide range of practices that train the mind to focus and cultivate specific qualities, such as calmness, concentration, and compassion. Some common meditation techniques include:

   - Concentration Meditation: Focusing attention on a single object, like the breath or a mantra, to achieve mental clarity and calmness.
   - Loving-Kindness Meditation: Cultivating feelings of love, compassion, and goodwill toward oneself and others.
   - Body Scan Meditation: Gradually bringing attention to different parts of the body,

promoting relaxation and body awareness.

- Transcendental Meditation (TM): Using a specific mantra to achieve deep relaxation and promote inner peace.
- Mindfulness-Based Stress Reduction (MBSR): An eight-week program that combines mindfulness meditation with yoga and body awareness techniques to reduce stress and improve overall well-being.

Benefits of Mindfulness and Meditation Practices:

1. Stress Reduction: Mindfulness and meditation practices can activate the body's relaxation response, reducing stress and anxiety levels.
2. Improved Focus and Concentration: Regular practice can enhance concentration, attention span, and cognitive abilities.
3. Emotional Regulation: Mindfulness practices help individuals become more aware of their emotions and develop healthier ways of responding to them.
4. Enhanced Self-Awareness: By cultivating non-judgmental self-awareness, individuals gain insights into their thought patterns and behaviors.
5. Better Sleep: Mindfulness and meditation can help improve sleep quality and reduce insomnia.
6. Pain Management: Mindfulness-based techniques have been used effectively to manage chronic pain and improve overall pain tolerance.
7. Increased Resilience: Regular practice can foster resilience and coping skills, helping individuals navigate challenges more effectively.

Mindfulness and meditation practices are generally safe and can be incorporated into daily life. They are adaptable and can be practiced individually or as part of structured programs and classes. Consistency and regularity in practice yield the most significant benefits. As with any new practice, it may take time to build familiarity and comfort, but over time, individuals often find these techniques profoundly beneficial for their mental, emotional, and even physical well-being.

Osteopathy

Osteopathy is a form of alternative or complementary medicine that focuses on the diagnosis and treatment of musculoskeletal disorders and their impact on the overall health of the body. It was founded by Andrew Taylor Still in the late 19th century and is based on the principle that the body has the innate ability to heal itself if given the right conditions.

Key Principles of Osteopathy:

1. Holistic Approach: Osteopathy views the body as a whole, interconnected unit. Practitioners consider the relationships between different body systems and structures when diagnosing and treating conditions.
2. Structure and Function: Osteopaths believe that the structure of the body influences its function, and vice versa. They aim to restore balance and alignment to the musculoskeletal system to improve overall health and well-being.
3. Hands-on Treatment: Osteopathic physicians use manual techniques, such as manipulation, mobilization, and massage, to diagnose and treat conditions. They focus on manipulating the body's tissues, including muscles, bones, ligaments, and fascia, to facilitate healing and restore optimal function.
4. Emphasis on Self-Healing: Osteopathy emphasizes the body's ability to heal itself, and practitioners aim to support and enhance this natural healing process.
5. Prevention: Osteopaths believe in preventing health issues by promoting overall well-being and providing advice on lifestyle, nutrition, and exercise.

Conditions Treated by Osteopathy: Osteopathy is commonly used to address a wide range of musculoskeletal problems, including:

- Back pain
- Neck pain
- Joint pain and stiffness
- Headaches and migraines
- Postural problems
- Sports injuries
- Arthritis
- Repetitive strain injuries

Osteopathic Treatment Techniques: Osteopathic treatment typically involves a range of manual techniques, such as:

- Soft tissue manipulation: Stretching and applying pressure to muscles, tendons, and ligaments to relieve tension and improve circulation.
- Joint mobilization: Gently moving joints within their normal range of motion to improve flexibility and reduce stiffness.
- High-velocity, low-amplitude (HVLA) manipulation: Quick, controlled movements to restore joint function and alignment.
- Myofascial release: Applying gentle pressure to the fascia, the connective tissue surrounding muscles, to release tension and improve mobility.
- Craniosacral therapy: Gentle manipulation of the skull and spine to address imbalances in the craniosacral system and promote relaxation.

Scope of Practice: Osteopathy is practiced by licensed professionals known as osteopaths or osteopathic physicians, depending on the country. They undergo extensive training and education in anatomy, physiology, pathology, and manual techniques to provide safe and effective care.

It is essential to note that osteopathy is a regulated healthcare profession in many countries, and practitioners are required to adhere to professional standards and ethical guidelines.

Overall, osteopathy is a non-invasive and drug-free approach to healthcare that aims to promote natural healing, restore balance, and improve overall health and well-being. It can be used in combination with conventional medical treatments or as an alternative therapy, depending on the individual's needs and preferences.

Principles and philosophy of osteopathic medicine

The principles and philosophy of osteopathic medicine are based on a holistic approach to healthcare, focusing on the interconnectedness of the body's systems and its innate ability to heal itself. Osteopathic medicine shares many principles with traditional medicine, but it also incorporates unique concepts that guide its practice. These principles are:

1. The Body is a Unit: Osteopathic medicine views the human body as a unified and interconnected entity. All body systems are interrelated and function together as a whole. Any dysfunction in one part of the body can have an impact on other areas.

2. Structure and Function are Interrelated: Osteopathic physicians believe that the structure of the body influences its function and vice versa. A balanced musculoskeletal system is essential for optimal health and well-being. Osteopaths use manual techniques to restore balance and alignment, which can improve overall function and promote healing.

3. The Body Has Self-Healing Mechanisms: Osteopathic medicine acknowledges the body's inherent ability to heal itself. Osteopaths aim to support and enhance this natural healing process by removing obstacles to recovery and providing appropriate conditions for healing.

4. Rational Treatment: Osteopathic physicians use a scientific and evidence-based approach to diagnose and

treat medical conditions. They consider the patient's medical history, physical examination, and relevant diagnostic tests to develop a comprehensive treatment plan.

5. Prevention: Osteopathic medicine emphasizes the importance of preventive healthcare. Osteopaths work with patients to identify risk factors and promote healthy lifestyle choices to prevent illness and optimize well-being.

6. Treatment of the Person, Not the Disease: Osteopathic medicine takes into account the individuality of each patient. Osteopaths consider the physical, emotional, and social aspects of a person's life when formulating a treatment plan. They view the patient as a whole person, not just a collection of symptoms.

7. Osteopathic Manipulative Treatment (OMT): OMT is a core aspect of osteopathic medicine. It involves hands-on techniques to diagnose and treat musculoskeletal issues, improve joint mobility, and alleviate pain. OMT can complement other medical treatments or be used as a standalone therapy, depending on the patient's needs.

8. Physician as a Partner in Health: Osteopathic physicians see themselves as partners in their patients' health journey. They strive to educate and empower patients to take an active role in managing their health and making informed decisions about their well-being.

Osteopathic medicine is recognized as a distinct healthcare profession in many countries, and osteopathic physicians complete rigorous training and education to become licensed practitioners. They are qualified to diagnose and treat medical conditions, prescribe medications, and perform surgery if necessary.

Overall, the principles and philosophy of osteopathic medicine reflect a patient-centered approach to healthcare, promoting the body's natural healing abilities and recognizing the interconnectedness of all aspects of health and well-being.

Osteopathic manipulative techniques and bodywork

Osteopathic manipulative techniques (OMT) are a key component of osteopathic medicine, involving hands-on therapeutic approaches to diagnose, treat, and prevent musculoskeletal issues and other medical conditions. OMT is used to restore balance, improve joint mobility, enhance circulation, and alleviate pain. Osteopathic physicians, also known as Doctors of Osteopathy (DOs), employ various manipulative techniques and bodywork to achieve these goals. Some common OMT techniques include:

1. Soft Tissue Techniques: These techniques target muscles, tendons, ligaments, and other soft tissues to release tension and promote relaxation. Examples include myofascial release, soft tissue stretching, and muscle energy techniques.
2. Joint Mobilization: Joint mobilization involves gentle and controlled movements to improve joint flexibility and restore normal range of motion. Techniques may include traction, compression, and passive joint movements.
3. Muscle Energy Technique (MET): MET is a form of stretching and relaxation that involves the patient's active participation. The patient contracts a specific muscle while the osteopath provides resistance, followed by relaxation and passive stretching.
4. High-Velocity Low-Amplitude (HVLA) Thrust: This technique involves quick and controlled movements of a joint beyond its passive range of motion. It is commonly

used for joint adjustments, particularly in the spine.

5. Counterstrain Technique: This method involves placing the patient's affected body part in a comfortable position to relieve muscle tension and pain. The goal is to reset the muscle's reflexes and promote healing.

6. Craniosacral Therapy: This gentle technique focuses on the craniosacral system, which includes the skull, spine, and cerebrospinal fluid. The osteopath uses light touch to assess and release restrictions in the craniosacral system.

7. Visceral Manipulation: Visceral manipulation targets the internal organs to improve their mobility and function. It can be beneficial for conditions related to organ dysfunction or post-surgical adhesions.

8. Lymphatic Pump Techniques: These techniques aim to improve lymphatic circulation and drainage, which can help reduce swelling and enhance the immune response.

OMT is tailored to each patient's specific needs and condition. Osteopathic physicians use their hands to palpate and assess the body's structures, identifying areas of restriction or dysfunction. The gentle, hands-on approach of OMT allows osteopaths to detect subtle changes in the body and address them before they lead to more significant issues.

OMT can be used as a standalone treatment or in conjunction with other medical interventions, depending on the patient's condition and needs. It is commonly used to treat musculoskeletal pain, back pain, neck pain, headaches, and various other conditions. The goal of OMT is to promote the body's natural healing processes, enhance overall well-being, and support the patient's health journey.

Conditions treated by osteopaths

Osteopaths, also known as Doctors of Osteopathy (DOs), are trained to diagnose and treat a wide range of medical conditions. They take a holistic approach to healthcare, focusing on the interconnectedness of the body's systems and the role of musculoskeletal health in overall well-being. Osteopathic physicians use osteopathic manipulative techniques (OMT) along with traditional medical treatments to address various health conditions. Some of the conditions commonly treated by osteopaths include:

1. Musculoskeletal Pain: Osteopaths are particularly skilled in treating musculoskeletal issues, including back pain, neck pain, joint pain, and sports injuries.
2. Headaches and Migraines: OMT can help relieve tension in the head, neck, and shoulders, which may contribute to headaches and migraines.
3. Postural Problems: Osteopaths can address postural imbalances and alignment issues that may lead to chronic pain or discomfort.
4. Osteoarthritis: OMT can help improve joint mobility and reduce pain in individuals with osteoarthritis.
5. Respiratory Conditions: Osteopaths can assist with conditions such as asthma and chronic obstructive pulmonary disease (COPD) by addressing musculoskeletal factors that impact breathing.
6. Digestive Disorders: OMT may benefit individuals with digestive issues like irritable bowel syndrome (IBS) by addressing tension in the abdomen and improving organ function.

7. Repetitive Strain Injuries: Osteopaths can provide relief for injuries resulting from repetitive motions, such as carpal tunnel syndrome.
8. Pregnancy-Related Pain: OMT can help ease pregnancy-related musculoskeletal pain, including lower back pain and pelvic discomfort.
9. Post-surgical Rehabilitation: Osteopaths can support recovery after surgery by promoting proper healing and addressing musculoskeletal imbalances.
10. Sports Injuries: Osteopaths often work with athletes to address sports-related injuries and optimize performance.
11. Neurological Conditions: While osteopaths do not treat neurological disorders directly, OMT can assist in managing associated musculoskeletal symptoms and promoting overall well-being.
12. Stress and Anxiety: OMT can help reduce physical tension and stress, contributing to improved emotional well-being.

It is important to note that osteopaths work collaboratively with other healthcare professionals, and their treatments complement standard medical care. They take into account the patient's medical history, lifestyle, and individual needs to provide a personalized and comprehensive approach to treatment.

While osteopaths can address a wide range of conditions, they are not a substitute for specialized medical care in certain cases. Patients with specific medical concerns should seek appropriate medical attention from the relevant specialists. Osteopathic treatment can be used as part of an integrated approach to support overall health and well-being.

Integrating osteopathy with other alternative therapies

Integrating osteopathy with other alternative therapies can enhance the effectiveness of treatment and provide a more comprehensive approach to addressing health issues. Osteopathy, with its focus on the musculoskeletal system and the body's self-healing capabilities, can complement various alternative therapies. Some of the alternative therapies that can be integrated with osteopathy include:

1. Acupuncture: Combining osteopathy with acupuncture can provide a holistic approach to pain management and promote overall well-being. Acupuncture can help release energy blockages and promote healing, while osteopathy can address musculoskeletal imbalances that may contribute to pain.

2. Massage Therapy: Massage therapy and osteopathy share similarities in their focus on relieving muscle tension and promoting relaxation. Integrating both therapies can provide a more comprehensive treatment for musculoskeletal issues and stress-related conditions.

3. Chiropractic Care: Chiropractic adjustments and osteopathic manipulative techniques both aim to improve musculoskeletal alignment and nervous system function. Integrating these therapies can offer a more complete approach to spinal health and overall well-being.

4. Naturopathy: Osteopathy and naturopathy share a

holistic approach to healthcare. Combining both modalities can address not only musculoskeletal issues but also consider nutrition, lifestyle, and other factors that impact health.

5. Mind-Body Medicine: Integrating osteopathy with mind-body practices, such as meditation, yoga, and mindfulness, can help address both physical and emotional aspects of health. Mind-body practices can enhance the body's self-healing capabilities and promote overall balance.

6. Herbal Medicine: Some osteopaths may incorporate herbal medicine to support the body's healing process and address specific health concerns. Integrating herbal medicine with osteopathy can provide a more comprehensive approach to health and well-being.

7. Homeopathy: Homeopathy focuses on stimulating the body's natural healing responses through highly diluted remedies. Integrating osteopathy and homeopathy can provide a holistic approach to health and healing.

8. Reiki and Energy Healing: Reiki and other energy healing modalities can complement osteopathy by promoting energy flow and relaxation. Integrating these therapies can support the body's natural healing processes.

It is essential to work with healthcare professionals who are experienced in both osteopathy and the specific alternative therapies being integrated. Each individual's health needs and conditions are unique, so the treatment plan should be tailored to the patient's specific requirements.

Integrative approaches that combine osteopathy with other alternative therapies can be particularly beneficial for chronic pain management, stress reduction, and improving overall well-being. However, it is important to consult with qualified practitioners and medical professionals to ensure that the integrated approach is safe and appropriate for the individual's health condition.

Integrative Medicine

Integrative medicine is a holistic approach to healthcare that combines conventional medical practices with complementary and alternative therapies to promote overall well-being and address a wide range of health conditions. The field of integrative medicine emphasizes the partnership between the patient and healthcare provider, taking into account the individual's physical, emotional, mental, and spiritual aspects to create a personalized treatment plan.

Key principles of integrative medicine include:

1. Patient-Centered Care: Integrative medicine places the patient at the center of the care process. Practitioners take the time to listen to patients' concerns, understand their goals, and work collaboratively to develop a treatment plan that aligns with their unique needs.

2. Holistic Approach: Integrative medicine considers the whole person, not just their symptoms or medical condition. It takes into account physical, emotional, mental, and spiritual factors that influence health and well-being.

3. Combination of Modalities: Integrative medicine incorporates a variety of healing modalities, including conventional medicine, complementary therapies, and alternative treatments. These may include nutrition, herbal medicine, acupuncture, chiropractic care, mind-body practices, and more.

4. Focus on Prevention: Integrative medicine emphasizes preventive measures to maintain optimal health and reduce the risk of illness. This may involve lifestyle

changes, stress management, and health screenings.

5. Evidence-Based Practice: While integrative medicine explores various therapies, it also emphasizes the importance of evidence-based practices. Treatment decisions are made based on scientific research, clinical expertise, and patient preferences.

6. Collaboration Among Healthcare Providers: Integrative medicine encourages collaboration among healthcare providers from various disciplines. Practitioners work together to ensure comprehensive care and exchange information to benefit the patient's health.

7. Personalized Care Plans: Treatment plans in integrative medicine are tailored to each individual's unique needs and preferences. There is no one-size-fits-all approach, and patients are active participants in their healing journey.

Integrative medicine can be applied in various healthcare settings, including hospitals, clinics, and wellness centers. It is often used to complement conventional medical treatments, particularly in cases where patients seek to explore additional options for managing chronic conditions or improving overall well-being.

The field of integrative medicine continues to evolve, with ongoing research and growing recognition within the medical community. Many medical schools and institutions now offer training and programs in integrative medicine, promoting an integrated and patient-centered approach to healthcare. As more evidence emerges supporting the efficacy and benefits of integrative approaches, it is likely to become more widely accepted and integrated into mainstream healthcare practices.

The importance of collaboration between conventional and alternative medicine

Collaboration between conventional and alternative medicine is crucial for several reasons, as it can lead to improved patient outcomes, enhanced healthcare options, and a more comprehensive approach to healing. Here are some key reasons highlighting the significance of such collaboration:

1. Holistic Patient Care: Integrating conventional and alternative medicine allows healthcare providers to consider the whole person, addressing not just physical symptoms but also emotional, mental, and spiritual aspects of health. This holistic approach can lead to more effective and well-rounded treatment plans.

2. Personalized Treatment: Each patient is unique, and what works for one individual may not work for another. By collaborating and combining different approaches, healthcare providers can create personalized treatment plans that align with the patient's preferences and needs.

3. Comprehensive Healthcare: Alternative medicine can offer valuable treatment options that may not be available in conventional medicine. Collaborating with alternative medicine practitioners provides patients with a broader range of healthcare choices, expanding the possibilities for addressing their health concerns.

4. Managing Chronic Conditions: For patients with chronic conditions that may not respond well to conventional treatments alone, alternative therapies can complement

and enhance the effectiveness of standard care, improving symptom management and overall quality of life.

5. Reducing Side Effects: Some conventional medical treatments can be associated with significant side effects. Integrating alternative therapies can help manage these side effects and improve the patient's overall well-being during treatment.

6. Prevention and Wellness: Alternative medicine often emphasizes prevention and lifestyle changes, promoting overall wellness and reducing the risk of certain health conditions. Collaborating with alternative medicine practitioners can strengthen a patient's focus on prevention and long-term health.

7. Patient Satisfaction: Collaborative care that respects the patient's choices and preferences can lead to higher patient satisfaction, which, in turn, may positively impact treatment adherence and overall health outcomes.

8. Evidence-Based Practice: By collaborating, conventional and alternative medicine practitioners can share knowledge, research, and evidence-based practices, fostering a more informed and evidence-driven approach to healthcare.

9. Health Education: Integrating alternative medicine into conventional settings can lead to greater awareness and understanding of different healing modalities among healthcare professionals and the public.

10. Bridging the Gap: Collaboration helps bridge the gap between conventional and alternative medicine, promoting better communication, mutual respect, and a more unified approach to patient care.

It's important to note that collaboration between conventional and alternative medicine should be based on mutual respect and open communication. Healthcare providers from both disciplines should be willing to share information and work together for the benefit of the patient. Integrative medicine, which combines both conventional and alternative therapies, is an example of a healthcare model that aims to achieve such collaboration and provide the best possible care to patients.

The rise of integrative medical centers and clinics

The rise of integrative medical centers and clinics is a response to the growing interest in holistic and patient-centered healthcare. Integrative medicine combines conventional medical treatments with evidence-based alternative therapies, aiming to address the physical, emotional, mental, and spiritual aspects of health. Several factors have contributed to the increasing popularity of integrative medical centers and clinics:

1. Demand for Holistic Care: Patients are increasingly seeking healthcare that goes beyond just addressing physical symptoms. They want a more comprehensive approach that considers their overall well-being and lifestyle factors.
2. Focus on Prevention: Integrative medicine places a strong emphasis on preventive care and lifestyle changes, promoting wellness and reducing the risk of chronic diseases.
3. Growing Awareness of Alternative Therapies: As the public becomes more aware of alternative therapies and their potential benefits, there is a demand for integrating these therapies with conventional treatments.
4. Supportive Research: The growing body of research supporting the effectiveness of some alternative therapies has increased the credibility of integrative medicine.
5. Patient-Centered Approach: Integrative medical centers

and clinics often prioritize the patient's preferences, needs, and values, involving them in the decision-making process and creating personalized treatment plans.

6. Multidisciplinary Collaboration: Integrative medical centers bring together healthcare providers from various disciplines, encouraging collaboration and sharing of expertise.

7. Improved Patient Outcomes: Integrative medicine has shown promising results in improving patient outcomes, especially for chronic conditions where conventional treatments alone may not be sufficient.

8. Cost-Effectiveness: Integrative medicine can potentially reduce healthcare costs by focusing on prevention and reducing the need for more expensive medical interventions.

9. Addressing Chronic Pain and Mental Health: Integrative medicine is often sought after for managing chronic pain and addressing mental health conditions, as it offers a broader range of treatment options.

10. Shift in Healthcare Paradigm: The shift towards patient-centered care and a focus on overall wellness aligns with the principles of integrative medicine.

Integrative medical centers and clinics typically offer a variety of services, including acupuncture, chiropractic care, naturopathy, mind-body medicine, nutrition counseling, and more. These centers provide a supportive environment where patients can explore a combination of treatments tailored to their specific needs. Integrative medicine continues to gain momentum, and its growth reflects the evolving healthcare landscape's focus on holistic, personalized, and evidence-based approaches to health and well-being.

Case studies showcasing successful integration of modalities

Case Study 1: Managing Chronic Pain with Integrative Approach

Patient Profile: Sarah, a 45-year-old woman with chronic lower back pain.

Background: Sarah had been experiencing persistent lower back pain for several years, which was affecting her daily life and overall well-being. She had tried various conventional treatments, including medications and physical therapy, but the pain remained unresolved.

Integrative Approach:

1. Chiropractic Care: Sarah started receiving regular chiropractic adjustments to correct spinal misalignments and improve joint mobility in her lower back.
2. Acupuncture: Acupuncture sessions were introduced to help alleviate pain, reduce inflammation, and promote relaxation.
3. Mind-Body Techniques: Sarah learned relaxation and mindfulness techniques to manage stress, which can exacerbate pain perception.
4. Physical Therapy: The integrative team collaborated with a physical therapist to design a personalized exercise program focused on strengthening core muscles and improving posture.

Results: After a few weeks of integrative treatment, Sarah

reported significant improvement in her lower back pain. The combination of chiropractic adjustments, acupuncture, mind-body techniques, and targeted exercise contributed to her pain reduction and enhanced quality of life.

Case Study 2: Anxiety Management with an Integrative Approach

Patient Profile: John, a 30-year-old man struggling with anxiety and panic attacks.

Background: John had been experiencing frequent anxiety symptoms, including racing thoughts, heart palpitations, and difficulty sleeping. He wanted to explore non-medication options for managing his anxiety.

Integrative Approach:

1. Cognitive Behavioral Therapy (CBT): John began working with a licensed therapist trained in CBT to identify and modify thought patterns contributing to his anxiety.
2. Mindfulness Meditation: John learned mindfulness meditation techniques to increase present-moment awareness and reduce anxiety-related rumination.
3. Herbal Medicine: An herbalist recommended specific herbs known for their calming effects, such as chamomile and passionflower, to support John's nervous system.
4. Nutritional Counseling: A nutritionist provided guidance on dietary changes, including reducing caffeine and increasing nutrient-dense foods to support mental well-being.

Results: After several weeks of integrative treatment, John reported reduced anxiety levels, better sleep, and improved overall mood. The combination of CBT, mindfulness meditation, herbal support, and dietary adjustments contributed to his progress in managing anxiety.

Case Study 3: Integrative Cancer Care

Patient Profile: Linda, a 55-year-old woman diagnosed with breast cancer.

Background: Linda was undergoing conventional cancer treatments, including surgery, chemotherapy, and radiation. However, she wanted to complement her medical treatments with integrative therapies to support her overall well-being and coping with side effects.

Integrative Approach:

1. Nutritional Support: A registered dietitian worked with Linda to develop a nutrition plan that focused on maintaining adequate nutrient intake during treatment and supporting her immune system.
2. Mind-Body Therapies: Linda participated in yoga and meditation classes to reduce stress, enhance relaxation, and improve her emotional well-being.
3. Massage Therapy: Regular massage sessions were incorporated to alleviate muscle tension and improve circulation.
4. Supportive Counseling: A licensed counselor provided emotional support and coping strategies to help Linda navigate the emotional challenges of her cancer journey.

Results: Linda found that the integrative approach helped her manage side effects from conventional treatments and cope better with the emotional aspects of her cancer diagnosis. She felt more empowered and supported throughout her cancer journey.

These case studies demonstrate the successful integration of various modalities within an integrative approach to healthcare. Each patient's treatment plan was tailored to their unique needs, highlighting the importance of personalized and holistic care in achieving positive outcomes. Integrative medicine can be a valuable complement to conventional treatments, addressing the physical, emotional, and spiritual aspects of health to support overall well-being and enhance quality of life.

Future trends in alternative and holistic medicine

The field of alternative and holistic medicine is continuously evolving to meet the changing needs and preferences of patients. Some future trends in this area include:

1. Increased Integration with Conventional Medicine: As more research supports the efficacy of certain alternative therapies, there will likely be increased integration of these modalities with conventional medicine. Collaborative care models that combine the best of both approaches can offer comprehensive and personalized treatment plans for patients.

2. Digital Health and Telemedicine: Technology is transforming healthcare delivery, and alternative and holistic medicine is no exception. Telemedicine and digital health platforms are making it easier for patients to access alternative therapies remotely, receive virtual consultations, and access wellness programs.

3. Personalized Medicine: The future of healthcare is moving towards personalized treatment plans tailored to an individual's unique needs and genetic makeup. In alternative and holistic medicine, personalized medicine will focus on identifying therapies and lifestyle interventions that work best for each patient.

4. Mind-Body Therapies: The recognition of the mind-body connection in health and wellness is growing. Mind-body therapies like meditation, yoga, and mindfulness are likely to gain more acceptance and use in

mainstream healthcare settings.

5. Evidence-Based Practices: As alternative and holistic medicine gains more recognition, there will be increasing demand for evidence-based practices. Research studies and clinical trials will help establish the effectiveness of various alternative therapies and guide their integration into healthcare systems.

6. Focus on Preventive Care: With a growing emphasis on preventive care, alternative and holistic medicine will play a vital role in promoting wellness and addressing the root causes of health issues before they become chronic.

7. Wellness Tourism: As more individuals seek holistic approaches to health, wellness tourism, which involves traveling to destinations that offer alternative therapies and wellness programs, is expected to increase.

8. Herbal Medicine and Natural Supplements: With a growing interest in natural and plant-based remedies, herbal medicine and natural supplements are likely to become more popular as people seek alternatives to pharmaceuticals.

9. Integrative Cancer Care: Integrative approaches to cancer care, combining conventional treatments with complementary therapies to support patients' overall well-being, are gaining traction and are expected to continue to evolve.

10. Mental Health and Holistic Practices: As mental health issues become more prevalent, the integration of holistic practices, such as mindfulness-based therapies and art therapy, into mental health treatment plans is likely to expand.

Overall, the future of alternative and holistic medicine is promising, with increasing recognition, integration, and evidence-based practices that support patients' well-being and enhance the overall healthcare landscape.

Recap of key insights and learnings

Throughout our discussion on alternative and holistic medicine, we explored various modalities and approaches that focus on treating the whole person – mind, body, and spirit. Here are some key insights and learnings from our conversation:

1. Holistic Approach: Alternative and holistic medicine emphasizes the interconnectedness of physical, emotional, mental, and spiritual well-being. It considers each individual as a unique entity with their own health needs.

2. Naturopathy: Naturopathic medicine emphasizes the body's innate ability to heal itself and uses natural therapies like herbal medicine, homeopathy, and hydrotherapy to support healing.

3. Acupuncture: Based on Traditional Chinese Medicine, acupuncture aims to balance the body's energy flow through meridians to promote healing and alleviate various conditions.

4. Chiropractic: Chiropractors focus on the spine's alignment and the nervous system's function to support overall health and treat musculoskeletal conditions.

5. Mind-Body Medicine: The mind-body connection is crucial in health and disease. Techniques like meditation, mindfulness, and hypnotherapy can positively impact overall well-being.

6. Diet Therapy: Nutrition plays a significant role in promoting health and preventing diseases. Specific diets can be tailored to address various health conditions.

7. Osteopathy: Osteopathic medicine emphasizes the

musculoskeletal system's importance in overall health and uses manipulative techniques to promote healing.

8. Integrative Medicine: Integrative medicine combines conventional and alternative approaches to create comprehensive and personalized treatment plans for patients.

9. Collaboration and Personalization: The future of healthcare lies in collaboration, evidence-based practices, and personalized treatment plans that cater to individual needs.

10. Wellness and Preventive Care: Holistic medicine focuses on promoting wellness and preventing diseases by addressing root causes and lifestyle factors.

11. Patient-Centered Care: The patient's needs, values, and preferences are central to alternative and holistic medicine.

12. Ethical Considerations: Practitioners in these fields must adhere to ethical guidelines and prioritize patient safety and informed consent.

13. Research and Evidence: As alternative and holistic medicine gains recognition, more research and evidence-based practices are emerging to support their effectiveness.

14. Wellness Tourism: The rise of wellness tourism reflects the growing interest in seeking alternative therapies and wellness experiences.

Overall, alternative and holistic medicine provides a comprehensive and patient-centered approach to healthcare, recognizing the importance of addressing the whole person for optimal well-being. By integrating conventional and complementary therapies, practitioners can create effective and individualized treatment plans to support patients' overall health and quality of life.

Emphasizing the value of Alternative & Holistic Medicine in modern healthcare

Alternative and holistic medicine has gained increasing recognition and value in modern healthcare for several reasons:

1. Personalized Approach: Alternative and holistic medicine treats individuals as unique beings with individual health needs. It emphasizes personalized treatment plans, considering all aspects of a person's health – physical, emotional, mental, and spiritual.

2. Focus on Prevention: These modalities prioritize preventive care and wellness promotion, aiming to address underlying causes of health issues rather than just treating symptoms. This approach can lead to better long-term health outcomes.

3. Patient-Centered Care: Alternative and holistic medicine puts the patient at the center of the treatment process. Practitioners take the time to understand their patients' needs, values, and preferences, fostering a more compassionate and collaborative healthcare experience.

4. Integrative Care: By integrating conventional medical treatments with complementary therapies, healthcare providers can offer comprehensive care that addresses a wide range of conditions and enhances patients' overall well-being.

5. Mind-Body Connection: Recognizing the intricate relationship between the mind and body, these modalities harness the power of the mind's influence on physical health. Techniques like meditation,

mindfulness, and hypnotherapy can complement traditional treatments and improve patient outcomes.

6. Empowerment and Self-Care: Alternative and holistic medicine empowers individuals to take an active role in their health through lifestyle changes, dietary modifications, and self-care practices, promoting a sense of responsibility for one's well-being.

7. Holistic Healers: Practitioners in these fields often spend more time with patients, allowing for deeper discussions and comprehensive assessments. They focus on nurturing the doctor-patient relationship, which can positively impact patient satisfaction and adherence to treatment plans.

8. Natural and Low-Risk Therapies: Many alternative therapies, such as herbal medicine and dietary changes, have a lower risk of adverse effects compared to some conventional treatments. This makes them attractive options for individuals seeking less invasive and more natural approaches.

9. Supporting Chronic Conditions: Alternative and holistic therapies can be valuable in managing chronic conditions that may not have complete cures in conventional medicine. They can improve quality of life and symptom management for patients with long-term health challenges.

10. Expanding Research and Evidence: As interest in alternative and holistic medicine grows, more research is being conducted to validate the efficacy of various modalities. Evidence-based practices contribute to the credibility and integration of these therapies in modern healthcare.

Incorporating alternative and holistic medicine into modern healthcare can lead to more comprehensive, patient-centered, and effective approaches to treating a diverse range of health conditions. As we continue to explore and understand the value of

these modalities, they will play an increasingly important role in shaping the future of healthcare.

Encouragement to explore and embrace alternative approaches to health and healing

Embracing alternative approaches to health and healing can be a transformative journey that opens up new possibilities for your well-being. Here's some encouragement to explore and embrace these modalities:

1. Personal Empowerment: By exploring alternative approaches, you take an active role in your health and well-being. You become empowered to make informed decisions and tailor your healing journey to suit your unique needs.
2. Holistic Care: Alternative therapies consider your whole being – mind, body, and spirit. This holistic approach addresses not just symptoms but the root causes of health imbalances, leading to comprehensive healing.
3. Complementing Conventional Medicine: Integrating alternative therapies with conventional medicine can enhance your overall treatment plan. It may improve treatment outcomes, reduce side effects, and support faster recovery.
4. Individualized Solutions: Alternative approaches recognize that everyone's health journey is different. They offer personalized solutions that consider your lifestyle, preferences, and values.
5. Safe and Natural Options: Many alternative therapies use natural elements and gentle techniques, minimizing the risk of adverse effects. They can be especially beneficial for those seeking non-invasive and drug-free

options.

6. Stress Reduction: Mind-body practices like meditation, mindfulness, and yoga can reduce stress and promote relaxation, benefiting your physical and mental health.

7. Empathy and Compassion: Alternative practitioners often prioritize building strong patient-practitioner relationships. Their empathetic and compassionate care can create a nurturing healing environment.

8. Treating Chronic Conditions: Alternative therapies can offer support for chronic conditions that may not have complete cures. They can improve symptoms, manage pain, and enhance overall quality of life.

9. Prevention and Wellness: Alternative medicine focuses on preventive care, helping you maintain your health and prevent future health challenges.

10. Expanding Perspectives: Exploring alternative approaches introduces you to diverse healing traditions from different cultures, broadening your understanding of health and well-being.

Remember, alternative approaches are not meant to replace conventional medicine but to complement it. Always consult with healthcare professionals and seek evidence-based practices. Embracing alternative approaches can be a beautiful journey of self-discovery and healing, guiding you toward a more balanced and vibrant life. It's an invitation to embrace your own agency and explore the full spectrum of health and healing possibilities available to you.